Introducing Women's Self Defence

Introducing Women's Self Defence

Covering Mindset, Techniques and Tactics To Get You One Step Ahead

50+ Master Lessons In Self Defence
That Every Woman And Girl Needs To Know

By Hafiz Younis

Chief Coach at **Power For Women** Self defence
BSc (Hons) Sport Science
Former Met Police Officer
British Combat Association Instructor

COPYRIGHT

SPECIAL INFORMATION

Please allow me to mention that we have tailored courses for corporates, education institutions and individuals. You can contact us with the email below or mention us to your gender network, DEI or welfare lead or other appropriate person.

We can pop to your place to deliver skills to you directly and personally.

For enquiries please contact me at:
www.power-for-women.org/enquiries
We can't wait to help you.

Hafiz Younis + Power For Women team.

WE HAVE MORE BOOKS AND COURSES!
Please check us out at www.power-for-women.org and follow the relevant links

Thank you.

DEDICATION

This book is dedicated to my mother and sisters and nieces and female friends and anyone else like them who doesn't need and doesn't deserve the hassle they get from too many men. The world changes and hopefully one day you will all face less of this unnecessary trauma. Some men should know better but until that time you might need to kick them in the you-know-what to get some sense into them. This book will help you do that.

Acknowledgements. I would like to thank two specific angels the most. They came in the form of school teachers, who would not let me stay in the gutter, no matter how hard I tried to stay there. Miss Hopewell and Mr Brown. My English teacher and my Biology teacher respectively. I don't even know your first names and you will never know how many times in life I have remembered you and thanked you. Without you I would never have left town, never would have got through school and most likely would have been in prison at some point, probably for violent crimes. You pushed me off that trajectory and I didn't see it until years went by. You went out of your way to do this. You didn't have to. Yet you did. And I will be grateful to you for that until the day I die. Maybe beyond.

I would also like to thank all those who pushed me, whether you meant to or not. Thank you to my friends and family and all the teachers on the way.

Thanks to Geoff Thompson for being a super massive inspiration in my life since the mid 1990s (and he doesn't even know it!)

Special thank you to Naveed Younis for editing this book late into the nights. Thanks also for your input to my brother Saeed Younis and sisters Rahilla, Kat and Aiysha, and my eldest nephew, Sahel Younis. Thank you to Natasha Lawrence for always being a rock of support.

TRIGGER WARNING/CAUTION

The subject matter within can be of a triggering nature, while at the same time this material needs to be accessible to all, including the younger readership and those who may already have suffered assaults. It would be unfair to not include that readership but also unfair to subject them to trauma they really could do without.

The idea of the book is to help develop a mindset and skillset, to get a deeply usable ability to defend yourself. It is difficult to achieve that if a lot of stressful and traumatic language and situations are mentioned consistently.

So for that reason I have kept the language accessible, so we can help as many women and girls as possible. However it would be unfair not to tackle sexual assault and therefore you can get this extra info at www.power-for-women.org/complement.

Note that everything in here is still as applicable to preventing and dealing with serious sexual assaults. It's just a few specific tactics have been left out.

Thereare some helpline numbers, towards the end of the book, for organisations that can help those who have been victims of violence or sexual assault, and other help too. So please do refer to these if you think they can help you. I have been lucky enough to have worked alongside some of these organisations and I can vouch they are generally very helpful and understanding of your situation. You do not need to suffer alone. Give them a call. They will help you in your time of need.

CONTENTS

DISCLAIMER

Before starting any of the training in here, please get clear instructions from a medical professional that you are okay to do the exercises, practices and anything else suggested in here. All physical training can lead to injury and it is your own personal duty to reduce the risks for yourself in all ways possible. Furthermore, should you use any of the advice or skills in this presentation it is again at your own risk. The author and all involved do not accept any liability for actions that stem from viewing this product or following any instructions or ideas from it. Everything is for information purposes only. If you are in any doubt then please do not copy any of the actions or any advice relayed in here. Please do not continue to view the product without taking this into consideration.

For under 18's we request you do not read nor apply this material without the explicit advice of a relevant authority, such as parent, guardian, the police, a lawyer and anyone else you are ensured is a correct and relevant authority to guide you.

What is contained in here is NOT legal advice of any kind. Our advice is to seek legal advice from a lawyer or others who are right for you to seek advice from. We do not endorse the use of these techniques or ideas. They are provided for information purposes only. All injuries serious or small, including death caused, is at your own risk.

This book does not represent the views or practices of any police service or group current or disbanded.

In short: do not participate in any suggested activities without first consulting the correct medical and legal professionals for your given circumstances.

PREFACE

Self defence is not martial arts. I have been doing both for about an eternity and it continues to grind me that people doing martial arts are led to believe they're doing self defence. There is cross-over, of course. Like you could use your LV handbag to carry your personal items or you could use it for carrying bricks when you're building a new wall in your garden. The hand//bag crosses over to do both jobs but it's not designed, nor suited, to do both jobs. It will do the job that it's designed for much better than the one you adapted it for.

Self defence and martial arts are exactly like that. They use the same or similar skills but to do two very different things.

The words 'martial arts' means the 'science of war'. 'Martial' stems from Mars, the god of war, and 'art' being used to mean study or science. It is great for soldiers and ninjas and assassins and those who have to stay to fight, to kill and be victorious.

Self defence is about getting away early, heading home to have tea and macarons and chill out with your friends.

Let's say you were inclined the martial way and only wanted to learn to kill. Which of the martial arts would you choose anyway? Is it kickboxing? Karate? Wu Shu?

They all show you how to stand up, kick and punch. But what if you get dragged to the floor?

Then must you learn jiu jitsu? Or is it wrestling? Maybe judo as well?

But... as a woman facing a man, do you really want to be fighting on the floor?

And how long do you want to train to become this assassin anyway? It takes about three years to become a black belt in most arts, not counting the financial costs and the pains and injuries you'll go through.

And you still didn't learn self defence because it is something other than becoming an assassin.

And as soon as a real self defence situations arises, you're going to find yourself quite lost.

How do I know this? Because I went through this process. To discover self defence, I drove through years and years figuring out what worked and what didn't. Back then, without the internet, you had to figure things for yourself. Martial arts were mystical and those who did them didn't reveal the secrets. They'd trained for decades to get their knowledge and they weren't going to spill the secrets just because you asked. You had to pay your dues in money, time, pain, devotion. And so I did. Karate and boxing, wrestling, judo and Brazilian jiu jitsu are the ones I've done most of, though I've dabbled in others too.

I had a deep need to know these because of where I grew up. How I grew up. To avoid violence, I had to know all about it. It became an obsession.

But it wasn't self defence.

Early on in my journey I was lucky enough to discover three coaches who at the time were starting to become legends in the martial arts world, and they had a skew towards self defence. So I learned everything I could from these three - Geoff Thompson, Peter Consterdine and Dave Turton - then reapplied what I'd already learned in the martial arts to self defence. It was a hard journey because everyone still said they were doing self defence when they were really doing martial arts, but I didn't need to learn how to bow deeply to my sensei or tie my kimono neatly so it didn't upset the referee, and I didn't need to learn the Japanese terms for the schoolboy's leg-trip throw (Osoto Gari, in case you're wondering!). I just needed to know what would save my skin when the poop smacked the wings of the fan.

I joined London's Metropolitan Police Service one day and I really did figure out what worked and didn't. I was pushed to test techniques every day, often several times a day. I spent years working the Leicester Square and Piccadilly areas, on Saturday nights, where my ability and resilience were tested against individuals and even against groups.

But the thing is I was a man fighting other men.

How would my three sisters fare in real life situations?

How would they do against a much bigger and stronger man?

I couldn't personally teach them as I lived two hundred miles away - and this was before the rise of the internet as a viable teaching tool so I couldn't teach them via video either.

So how would they protect themselves in this world? What martial art could they do?

The answer came over time, not an epiphany, but a gradual understanding. They had to do boxing, judo and jiu jitsu. That would cover all situations, from a standing point of view, being thrown and also how to deal with the floor. True, they'd be learning too many surplus skills in those arts, but the useful bits in them really are useful.

So that was it. That's what they'd do. And to complete their training I would advise them on the psychological aspects etc.

But guess what?

They didn't want to spend three years learning each of those! They had other things to do, apparently.

Better things to do than learning martial arts? Apparently, that's true! Some people don't want to spend decades learning martial arts. It was news to me.

So now I was personally committed to teaching my youngest sister (twenty years my junior), who was very keen and still just a child at the time. We did self defence 'things'…but did I mention she lived 200 miles away? Try organising training with someone living 200 miles away, who is still at school. It's not easy! But over the next decade or so we did make reasonable progression. Sometimes my other two sisters joined in too.

So I was lucky to be able to train my sister(s) and test my martial arts skills in the real world and see what worked and what didn't. I had enough knowledge that at one time I was verbally accepted to read a Masters degree in self defence studies at Manchester University. The head of the Master's programme really wanted to see me create a thesis from all my knowledge and get it published. But in the end the cost and commitment was too high. I'd have to leave my job and become a full time student for a few years and it was a little late in my lifecycle by then, I thought. That time had passed.

But I continued to apply that vast knowledge to teaching my sisters.

Something important dawned on me over this time. That all the self defence out there in the world is actually men's self defence - but women can go along and have a go at it.

Every situation coached out there was based around men attacking men. Men stand and challenge each other. It's an ego battle. You must stay and fight and win so your friends and family will know how tough you are. But I knew from police work that this was not what happened when women were attacked. They were ambushed or they were followed to start with, for example. Men's fights were in the open, with an audience usually. Women were attacked when they were alone and in more isolated locations.

The reasons that men fight are different to the reasons men attack women, and so their methodology - the modus operandi in police and legal jargon - was not alike. The psychology of the whole thing was different. The application of skills was different. Men and women have different strengths and weaknesses too so how can the same things apply for men as they do for women in self defence?

As I coached my sisters I had to adapt what we did from men's self defence needs to women's.

There was also a need to work on mindset. As I knew already, the Bad Guy always plays mind games and always uses trickery. He's a deceptive little git, there's not doubt. Even when it's a man against a man, the street-smart attacker will never play fair. This knowledge is severely lacking in the training of martial artists, who tend to find teeth knocked out in their first real encounter and wonder where it went wrong. It went wrong because you don't know about these people! You only know how to bow and fight fair. On the street you have to first neutralise the Bad Guy's trickery!

Funnily enough I'd coached pure self defence in some of London's prestigious health clubs but it was men's self defence I had been teaching to men and women, I now realised. So now I adapted what I knew and worked on the skills that would be most suitable for women and girls.

To cut the story short, I have been teaching physical activities and sports since I was 12 years old in the Royal Air Force cadets. That's where it all first started, and it has continued into a lifelong passion for me. However, when I joined the police I was not allowed to continue teaching self defence to civilians as it was considered a conflict of interest. I did train with and coach a few police officers but it was irregular and not official.

During this time I started putting together my notes into a comprehensive collection. Yes, I'm one of those people who makes too many notes on things and has files and files of paperwork that need to be collated some day.

So, when I left the police, when the first Covid lockdowns started, I had already begun putting a comprehensive course together for women's self defence. I wanted to craft something for my sisters (one of them had recently been robbed and badly affected by it) but I realised there was a greater need out there too and that this could be a great career change for me. I'd be combining my love of teaching sports and my deep understanding of martial arts and self defence. No one had actually differentiated between women's self defence, men's self defence and martial arts so this was something I was really keen to get done because it needed to be and I'd already started anyway. Now I wanted to be one of the first to teach things properly. And it seems there's never been a greater need for women's self defence in my lifetime as there is right now.

When covid bit hard I was already coaching a couple of women and I was invited by a major hight street bank's welfare officer to teach their female staff. They wanted online lessons that all their female staff could access and then I'd come along once a week for an online chat and review to iron out any issues they had. I was really looking forward to it…and then suddenly no one was at their workplace anymore! I also had a request from a local university and two private girls' schools but it was all put on hold at the same time. So I started to write this instead, to get my thoughts together, to make it easier to teach when I got back to it…and somehow it's turned into this book!

So I hope you enjoy this endeavour of mine. I know for a fact that you'll learn far more than you are bargaining for, learning the skills you genuinely need to mentally and physically take on any person who might try to harm you physically in one way or another.

I hope this book will exceed most of your expectations - and I also hope you never have to use anything in it either!

So, with my best regards, I warmly welcome you to enter this new world you have just discovered.

I will see you there.

Hafiz Younis

P.S. Whilst you read this, I'll hopefully be back to teaching - and not writing books! It's hard work all this writing malarkey and I might have to take my head off and send it on holiday somewhere to recover! I'm thinking Greece, Kefalonia. Any suggestions?

PART ONE:
INTRODUCING
WOMEN'S SELF DEFENCE

A MUST READ!

Self defence doesn't start with your fists. It starts with your head. Your brain to be precise. It's involved throughout the entire process even more than your fists are.

So why is self defence only coached as physical techniques?

Tactics and psychology play an equal part in defending yourself against any Bad Guy who wants to do you harm or take away your property. Self defence is not self defence if you don't know how to deal with your own mind and body AND his mind and body.

We're going to do that here in this book.

Just knowing a few techniques isn't good enough either. How to escape someone strangling you from behind is not good enough and learning just that is a disservice to yourself.

Why did you get into a strangle in the first place when there were at least seven or eight opportunities to have prevented that!

What are you doing getting strangled!

Of course, it can happen to anyone. We get ambushed. But the majority of attacks don't start that way, at the deep end. So why do self defence and the martial arts only teach how to get out of those deep situations? You could have avoided or escaped ages ago! You could have been home by now rather than fighting for your life!

That's what I'd rather be doing. I don't want to wait and let someone strangle me before I start doing self defence. Self defence starts with the mind, starts with avoidance. I want to beat this man at his game before he gets into it. I don't want to get into a physical altercation if I don't have to.

If you'd also rather be at home, with friends, munching macarons and drinking coffee (it's Victoria sponge and Harrod's Spiced Tea for me, thank you!) then this book is for you.

We are going to cover some amazing tactics here. Avoid, and if you can't, then defend early, escape early. Get away.

So, please allow me to quickly introduce what is coming your way.

In 'Part One: Introducing Women's Self defence' we will cover some elements you might be interested in, such as why this book is relevant to you plus a little bit of housekeeping so you know how to get through the book in a way best suited to you. This is a text-book and also a follow-along book. You can come back to it for reference purposes again and again. But you should also go through it and practice the skills. Many chapters have follow-along parts to them.

You need to have self defence in your head but you really should have it in your hands and feet too. You have to own the skills so they work when you need them.

The way the book is designed is to add layer upon layer of learning. There would be no point in giving you an info dump but then you have to figure it all out yourself. Instead of that we build a skill, and sometimes even a part of a skill, one bit at a time, add layers as we go along and add more layers. This way your understanding of women's self defence is going to be deeper. You will see how techniques link together and have the ability to apply them consistently and universally to many situations. Trust me, this was not easy to put together this way! It would have been much easier to stick some techniques before you and say, "There you go. Women's self defence. Do it yourself," then walk away. That's how it actually started but as I continued writing it felt like I was doing a disservice to the reader. What's the point of you knowing all those skills in your head but not being able to use them? So I changed it all so that if you follow along, you will get all the information that you need, but you will get many essential skills in your body and bones. Doing it this way ensures you progress and have skills developing at each stage.

In 'Part Two. Understanding the Bad Guy and Understanding Yourself' we cover the psychology that will help you survive. These principles are very important for your mindset. Read this section now, casually maybe. But come back to it and read it again a few times so you really know this information. In there is a lifetime of fighting psychology, fighting big guys and small guys. Some extremely violent. Some really tricky. Some who scared me and made every molecule in my body shake like apply jelly being electrocuted.

I have been involved in violence for so long and with so many people that I'm in a position to talk about it that is useful to you rather than in the ways an armchair enthusiast would do, which might be informative but of no practical use. My misfortune of a lifetime dealing with violent people comes to you as an advantage. We're going to do practical and useable psychology rather than textbook studies.

Can I just say though, in case you get the wrong message, I am not a violent person and never have been inclined to violence. It's just I've had a lifetime of having to deal with it. I've always intended to break away from it and never take part, but I also had to know what to do when it came my way. I just wanted to make it clear where I am coming from.

In 'Part Three: The Stages and Situations of Self defence' we start to now actually move into the situations and start actively learning the techniques. We start with the early stages. How to avoid situations before they get physical. How to deter an attacker or prevent him from even having a chance to grab us or hit us? You will learn practical skills that you can use right away to start protecting yourself this very day.

We then we progress into the deeper arenas and deal with the more severe situations and scenarios. Part Three is the longest section of the book as it covers all five stages of a self defence situation - covering skills you could use at home or at work, in a car park or the back of a van, whilst abroad on holiday or while walking home or being followed. Universal skills. There's even information on what to do after an incident.

There's a lot in this section but your job is to just follow along. Let me be your guide. That's my job.

Part Four is a brief section to make sure you see how the skills you've learned so far are applicable in so many situations. We quickly discuss the more common situations and locations you might want to deal with. We cover how to deal with someone who is following you for example. This is a unique tactic that you will not find anywhere else. A tactic I used to save myself many times as I patrolled the back streets of London alone at night

What did I do when someone was following me? You'll find out! It really is a great tactic.

'Part Five: Self defence Mastery' is the final section, where we cover The Magic Five. These are skills that take everything you've learned to a higher level. Each of these Magic Five is a super-enhancer of your skills. You can hit harder using these. You can push harder. You can pretty much do everything better. I know that's a massive claim and sounds preposterous, but just wait till you get there! You will literally be made stronger using these principles that I only normally reveal to those at the top end of being my students. But I had to add them here as it would have been unfair not to. I initially kept these out of the book but I'm glad I changed my mind and added them.

By the end of the book I hope you are a person transformed. I say that because that's what I've tried to do. I know it might appear a little big-headed of me but I genuinely want you to hold these skills and tactics in your feet and head, like I do. That should something happen you know what to do because it's all right there and you can use it to get home to safety.

If I can get anywhere near to achieving that then I will feel as if you and I have both succeeded and we are now a self defence team that Bad Guy won't like at all.

HOW TO BEST USE THIS BOOK

This is a practical follow-along book but you can also just read through.

There are many practical skills, which I encourage you to do either at the time of reading or soon after. Most of these are easy to follow. By doing them right away you will firstly be able to employ them right away and secondly you can move along to the next bit and keep progressing at a rapid rate. This way your skillset builds and continues to build up as you go through the book. One of the principles that I exist by is that every single lesson should be adding something to your overall ability AND be useable right away. One of the most annoying things I found in my decades of martial arts is that skills were coached almost randomly and it took years and years to figure out how things fitted together. It was like completing a giant jigsaw but the pieces were given to you absolutely randomly over many years. It literally wasted so much of my time doing it this way and I really had to avoid that for you. So it is not by chance that you are learning in this systematic way, it is by diligent design.

This book could have been the size of an encyclopaedia, easily, several volumes but I had to keep it readable. Nobody has time to read an encyclopaedia these days.

So it means that some things will be overviews rather than deep dives but there is more than enough for you to learn and to get you through most encounters you could face.

I believe this is quite a unique and important book. There is nothing else out there like it that will help you this way. It is the full works when you consider the psychological, physical and tactical elements it includes; to avoid situations all the way to surviving even vicious attacks. I think it is worth taking seriously.

So, you can read through the book from the start to the end. That works. No issues. The book has been done in a logical way to do that. Go through. Take notes. Or not. Do your thing.

That is probably the best way to go through it the first time. Maybe even have a five minute flick through the pages, familiarise yourself with the layout before you start. Then head in there and go from start to finish.

But you can also dip in and out. Go to the bits you want to know about right now. You might want to come back and keep working on a particular skill over time too.

The information is timeless. The techniques have longevity. They apply today, they will apply tomorrow and will continue to apply until the day men grow gills and a third arm. These skills won't change. Most of them are also applicable to any age that you are. Of course if you're at the extremes of age or wellness then you might struggle with some of these, but in general most women of most abilities should be able to work through these at their own pace. In the classes that I teach I have had people of all abilities, including some with physical disabilities, and we have worked around the skills and made them theirs. So just slow down or speed up. It's up to you.

PLEASE NOTE that Part One is an introduction to this book and to women's self defence in general.

It is not essential reading though is highly informative. The actual skills and training begin in Part Two so you can skip to that and come back later to read Part One if you prefer.

Just make sure you still read The First Two Rules Of Self defence if you're gong to skip ahead to Part Two.

If you want to skip you can do so from here. Or later. It's up to you.

It's your book, after all!

SOME THINGS YOU MIGHT LIKE TO KNOW BEFORE WE SET OFF

Let's quickly get a few things out of the way that will give you a better overview of what we're going to do here and why.

SO WHAT IS SELF DEFENCE?

Self defence is a legal and moral human right to protect yourself or another.

It is not the art of staying to fight. It is the art of avoidance first, escaping at every opportunity, and only fighting when you have to.

Firstly, walk away if you can. (But you were going to do that anyway, I know).

Secondly, escape, and keep escaping no matter what happens - whether you're only involved in a verbal discussion or the bad guy has fully grabbed you, get away as soon as you can. You'll find out how to do that throughout this book.

Thirdly, if you're forced to fight, then fight for your life. Do what you need to do to continue living. If that means you have to be very severe in your actions then you are morally obligated and legally allowed to do so.

This is what self defence is. It is not a 'fight'. You are not competing. There is no referee. It will not be a 'fair fight'.

And if you do fight, or you do hurt or kill someone, the law will question what you did as to the level and proportion of force that you used. But force is allowed all the way up to lethal force if you genuinely believe that you had to use it.

You have the right to defend yourself and your property.

(Note that the rules when protecting property are different to when protecting yourself but again proportionality applies. We won't be covering the defence of property here in this book. General advice with regards to property is to let the perpetrator have it and to then report it).

(Please seek legal advice for your country or region. The above is not legal advice in any way. It may or not apply in every country)

IS THERE A DIFFERENCE BETWEEN MEN'S AND WOMEN'S SELF DEFENCE?

Yes!

You knew that! You've probably always known that but maybe not exactly why.

Self defence is different for men and women.

As a woman you're not going to stand and exchange fisticuffs. Not against a man. Never in a million years will a man stand and face-off with you like in a martial arts movie or like you see in combat sports such as boxing.

That's never going to happen.

Attacks from behind, being grabbed, being pinned to the ground or a wall, being taken to the floor. Being dragged somewhere, or pushed somewhere. These are the things that women face.

These are not the things that men face primarily. Men usually stand in front of each other, for 90%+ of the time, and get ready to hit each other. That's how it starts.

A man attacking a woman is not the same. It's sneaky. The approach is from the rear or out of sight more often than not. The man usually wants to take control of the woman so the first thing he does is to grab her clothes, hair or wrists. He will then move her to the floor or a vehicle or at least a more secluded spot that he has pre-chosen. Any hitting he does is usually to further control the situation, to control the woman and not an ego-battle.

Men, in general, are stronger than women, and larger in size, and heavier. Their larger size gives them advantages in reach. Their extra strength means they can control a woman better and for longer (that won't be the case as you go through this book, I promise!). And the fact they are heavier means that they are more difficult to move around or move off you when they get on top. A woman is much easier to get off and easier to drag around or push about, in comparison.

This is just the start of the differences between women and men. There are many more and we can only have a women's self defence course if we start to deal with these quite huge differences in how the event unfolds and how the physicality varies.

To be able to get away from a man we have to know how to beat or neutralise the advantages he has.

We have to get an understanding of what tactics he will use so then we can start to get one step ahead of him.

HOW WILL I BE ONE STEP AHEAD OF THE ATTACKER?

Let's be straight here. You currently start one step behind when it comes to defending yourself, maybe even several steps behind. The attacker is usually prepared. Even if he is an opportunist, taking a chance rather than having things planned beforehand, he is likely to know the area better than you, and anyway, it's his decision to approach you, so he is one step ahead just because of that, to start with. If he's spent time scouting the location and knows where he can do his deed without getting spotted, and knows which way to run after, then we are several steps behind him already.

This is not like a jiu jitsu or combat sport competition. You won't be warmed up. You won't be mentally prepared for battle either or had time to study videos of your opponent so you can tackle him.

You do not start on an equal footing.

I don't want you to be on an equal footing. I actually want you to be one step ahead of what is going on in any self defence situation. At least one step. So this is another one of my Big Claims, right? I've already said I'm going to show you how to hit harder than you could ever imagine, and now I'm saying I'm going to get you one step ahead of an attacker? I'd better prove myself then otherwise you're going to fling this book at me!

So, how are we going to get one step ahead of someone who has the advantage on us when he starts?

There are several ways we are going to do this.

The very first thing is knowledge. By knowing all that can happen we can start to anticipate what might happen.

For example, there seem to be so many situations and scenarios that we could face in self defence. So many! They seem endless. It could be a car or a van that he jumps out of. It could be in the recreation park he appears from behind a tree. It could be the work or supermarket car park as we get in or exit our car. It could be on a beach when we're on holiday or a hotel room or a restaurant when going to the bathroom.

So many situations!

But that's not the case. If you think about it in each and every one of those scenarios there are only a finite number of things that can happen.

Let's say you've ended up on the floor. It doesn't matter too much if that floor is the floor of a restaurant bathroom, hotel bedroom or the back of a van or even on a bed. These are all situations where you are 'on the ground'. If you are on the 'ground' your fight plan remains pretty much the same. You do not need to study each of these locations individually. You can apply the same universal techniques and tactics to each of them.

Another way we get ahead of the situation is by understanding the methodology of attack. For example, in most situations there is an approach phase. The Bad Guy usually approaches you. (Ambush attacks are quite rare, luckily). Knowing this allows you to deal with him as he approaches rather than waiting until he's in touching distance right in front of you. (We will be using The Fence to do exactly this!).

There are a few more ways that we are going to get a step ahead of him but I'll mention only one important one here that I've found most instructors in self defence and martial arts don't seem to have figured out.

That is the use and development of universal skills.

My entire approach has always been to find the commonality amongst the skills I am learning. I don't want to learn ten thousand techniques. I want to learn one that covers five or ten or twenty situations. I want to know skills that apply across the board rather than specifically to one thing then never anywhere else. I've already said above that being on the floor is being on the floor for example. I've seen instructors teach how to get off the floor of a van, of a train carriage, of a bus, of a sandy beach and off a bed. They teach these individually as if each of them is so different. Yes, there are some *minor* variables with each but not enough to warrant learning them individually. Do you know how much time that would take anyway! The floor is the floor. If we covered every possible variable on earth for every possible situation, we would need two hundred lifetimes to learn it all. Which is about how long I've spent so far in my own life, and I don't see why you should also go through that process just 'because that's the way it is always done'.

Another example of a universally applicable skill is the Palm Heel. Most people teach how to punch, which, although is a great tool to own, is nowhere near as efficient nor as powerful nor as versatile as the Palm Heel, as you will soon discover. The Palm Heel can be used against a person taller than you or shorter. Or someone who is ducking down, or kneeling in front of you. It can be used on the floor to hit someone on the top of the skull if they managed to work their way between your legs. You can use it kneeling or standing and even lying down. You can't do all that with a punch.

And then there's the fact that punching is coached with gloves and wraps on. Do you know why? Because you'll break your hands if you punch a bag without them. What do you think will happen to your hand if you hit the hard skull of a man's face or head? Nobody ever tells you that you will break your bare hand the first time you punch a face hard. But it is really what happens. So how useful to you is a punch that breaks your hand the first or second time you blast is at a man? If you manage to stop him then it's been a very useful tool indeed, even if your hand breaks. But if you didn't stop him and you have to continue, now you only have one usable hand and the other one is in agony.

So I hope you are starting to see that we are going to cover some of the best techniques and tactics you will ever see, and you can also see how this relatively compact book really covers a vast amount of knowledge because of the way I have condensed it all for you.

Knowing that you have a handful of universally applicable skills that work, helps you to be one step ahead. You will know that these things work because you can actually try them out throughout the book.

And I'm going to keep suggesting that you practice these until you get tired of me saying it. Then I'll say it again one more time.

I don't want you to be one step ahead of him. I want you to be many steps ahead of him!!

WHERE AND HOW WOMEN ARE ATTACKED

Here are some of the most common things that women said to us in surveys, what they wanted to learn and what they were scared of. We'll cover these comprehensively and you will have the skills to deal with these (and much more!) by the end of the book.

These are their direct quotes:
"Do things and run away".
"Defend yourself in a high stress situation".
"Fear of being grabbed from behind or by the side when walking past bushes or an alleyway or a doorway".
"Being followed/walking alone at night".
"Getting into/out of car in a car park (in the dark)"
"Special tricks to defend yourself if someone was to attack you".
"Handle yourself in attempted mugging, violent attack or serious sexual assault or trying to grab you".
"Being at work late alone".
"Being attacked by a man much bigger than you who would be hard to fight off".
"I always get a bit panicky walking past a van in case the side door just opens and someone jumps out".

"Being pinned down".
"Staying alone in a hotel or AirBnB".
"Go for the soft spots in the event of an attack".
"Not knowing what to expect and worries about fitness and ability".

What is interesting about these comments is that they pretty much match the recorded data from the large organisations such as the UN WOMEN, the British Home Office, the FBI and the British police. So it appears that the fears are founded as they are shown by the recorded data of what actually happens.

We asked in the surveys why women hadn't started their self defence journey and these were some of the replies:
"Always putting it off. Always planned to do it, but never found time".
"Thought I wouldn't be able to do it because I'm too small and I would look stupid".
"Feels like now is the time in this scary world".
"Don't know where to even start looking for a class that is actually going to benefit me".
"You don't think it will happen to you until it does".

We then asked what might encourage them to follow a self defence programme:
"Must include at the information about how women are attacked differently to men".
"Avoid anything technical that is too hard to remember".
"Building confidence to defend yourself. If you're small you can feel intimidated by height and size of men"
"Include real life situations".
"Techniques using the other person's bodyweight against them".

Guess what? These are concerns that I've had myself too, since I was a child. These are the things that I was working towards finding solutions for when I first started my martial arts journey.

This book is based on research and statistics from UN WOMEN, the British Home Office, the FBI, the UK police, and other organisations too. With regards to what the stats say, most attacks in the UK (removing domestic assaults from this equation for the time being) occur on the street near the home - usually as you are on your way home in other words. Attacks are also prevalent inside the home (either your own or someone you know or have met recently). The other locations tend to be when going to a car or when leaving one (often car parks) and sometimes when leaving work.

That's what the stats show.

From my own experience of recording hundreds of robberies and attacks, I've seen them to occur mostly near public transport (usually when leaving a station or bus and heading home after work or an evening out). My own experience also shows that most altercations, or many of them, start either from the rear or from the sides - being blindsided quite often. Being followed, in other words, even for a short distance. I've discussed this with other officers and their experience also shows this to be the case, that most offences took place near public transport and at least half the time the approach was from the blind-side. However, this could also be skewed knowledge as everyone I spoke to worked in London, and most likely only ever in Westminster, which is where I worked the majority of my career.

So, being followed is something that is reported often but does not seem to appear in the published statistics, which also show that most attacks happen near the home but what I've seen in policing is attacks happen mostly near public transport.

Here are some other things you might like to know from the data.

The time of day or season is not as important as you might think. A more indicative factor is the location and the isolation of that location.

In other words attacks seem to occur more when you are away from people and less likely to be seen.

This is scary, of course, but it is something that you already knew anyway.

And we will actually use this to our advantage.

Consider the fact that most attacks on women occur in more isolated locations when there are very few people around. Why is this?

It's quite simple really. The attacker wants to get away with what he is doing.

They do not want to be caught. They do not want witnesses.

Another thing they usually want is to be speedy and that's for the same reason too. Even in cases of serious sexual assault, the man is usually quick about it. The data supports this. Of course there are times when that is not the case, but again these are rare instances.

What I'm trying to say is that this person is in a rush. And they don't want to be caught.

So what we want to do, our role during self defence, in essence, is to always try to disrupt everything they are doing. Delay them as much as we can, and make sure we are loud enough and physical enough that onlookers will call for help once they see we are in distress. Just the fact we are doing this from the very start means that it is more likely they will give up and leave, or else they will be caught.

In this book we are going to follow a tactic of deterring them, disrupting them and delaying them at every stage and at every single step along the way.

You will learn the skills to do this so that you automatically make things difficult for them to pursue.

For example we will be creating a stance/structure that stops them from being able to grab or hit us easily. But should he try, or even manage to actually grab you, the same stance disrupts him from moving you easily from one place to another. You will be drag-proof and push proof just by learning (practicing!) one single very effective way to stand, called The Fence.

Here's something else I didn't know until I started researching, But according to French studies, 75% of assaults on women occur in places where others are nearby. (https://www.cairn.info/revue-francaise- de-sociologie-1-2007-5-page-101.htm). That again means that being loud and obvious in what you're doing could alert others nearby. Whether you can see others nearby or not, it is very likely that someone is within earshot or might walk by at any time. So being loud and disrupting everything he does continues to be a great tactic to prevent escalation of a situation.

This report is worth a quick read. It adds that most assaults occur when you are moving from place to place, moving from one place to another on the street, or a parking lot, in a private vehicle, or on public transport.

It also says that 85% of the time the locations of attack were familiar to the women. In other words they had been there before and these were not places they had ventured into for the first time. That is also interesting to know because it means you can potentially move to a better location if you're currently isolated. You know the area where you are approached. Before he even approaches, you can start heading to a less isolated place or where there's CCTV or just a better chance of being seen.

So, I need to close this chapter off and make a point. Although the stats are very helpful in giving us an understanding and then creating some tactics to defend ourselves, the fact is that there is the real possibility that you might need to defend yourself anywhere and at any time. That's a fact. You knew it anyway and didn't need to hear it from me. But the reason I am mentioning it is not to scare you but so that you are not fixated on thinking you'll need self defence in the most common places shown by data. It can be a requirement to defend yourself anywhere.

But, for fear of repeating myself too much, that is why we are going to work on universal skills that can be applied in most, if not all, situations.

And these skills are tested, right? Yes! Tested in the real world. They work.

These are not just moves used in a dojo or fighting competition, these are psychological and physical skills and tactics that work in reality.

I'm not saying this for any other reason except that you should be confident in these skills working. They really are the real deal. Being confident in your actions means you will apply them with more determination and vigour and thus increase your chance of success multiple times. So you must believe in your ability.

I will make one more point with regards to where and how violence occurs.

Domestic violence is by far the most prevalent type of assault on women anywhere in the world. It has complex psychological and sociological aspects that I am not qualified to comment on and although we are not specifically going to cover domestic violence, I have dealt with hundreds of domestic violence situations in the police. More than hundreds if you count the perpetual domestic violence I grew up around. The thing is that, taking away the psychological aspects of domestic violence, without belittling what it is, the actual physical violence is the same as any other against a woman. So from that point of view the skills in this book are relevant to escape any domestic situation. Their application and psychological approach might be different but the skills that are in here work for all situations, as you will see. Whether you're being held on the floor by a stranger or a 'loved' one, the escapes are the same. I know the emotional elements are nowhere near the same, but the skills still do apply, and I genuinely hope they help some of the women out there who are subjected to this bilious and never-ending disease of domestic violence.

DO WE ALWAYS NEED TO USE DEADLY FORCE?

Yes. Absolutely.

You must always kill someone at every opportunity and every encounter.

That's a joke! Well, it's kind-of the martial arts and modern Krav Magaga view of self defence. Always choke them out or kill them in some way.

But in the really real world things are far more nuanced.

You can't just kill your co-worker when he attempts to kiss you beside the boiling kettle while you're waiting to make tea. Imagine the complaints from your work colleagues who take umbrage!

There are stages to everything in self defence. Just like 'going to work' has stages. You don't just get out of bed and go to work. You do many other things in between. Same applies to all self defence.

If you watched YouTube videos or went to jiu jitsu training you'll find that self defence starts when you're being strangled, are about to die and really need to survive and kill someone. And to do that, to kill them, even if they run away, you must hunt them down, fight to the death. Someone in class will grab you around the neck and tell you to escape. And once you've done that you've now done 'self defence' and can move on to the next move that's going to teach you how to kill or break arms.

So let's just go along with what they do. Let's say that in real life you were in a truly dangerous situation. Why and how did you get into that dangerous situation?!

Were there no strategies you could have employed which would have prevented you getting this far?

Yes! Of course, there were! You might have stopped the situation right at the start. You didn't have to wait until you were getting strangled. There were ten places at least you could have stopped all this escalation.

But, of course, regardless of what you do, you can still end up in deep trouble.

You're lying on an isolated beach in Italy, just sunning away when someone is right on you. You can be walking along the street in Marylebone in London after the bars shut and someone jumps from a dark doorway and is now strangling you. Or maybe a burglar has somehow got into your hotel room while you're in bed at night in the darkness. You thought the door was locked but it wasn't.

These are real examples I've investigated.

But they are very very rare. They do not happen often at all. That does not mean we won't prepare for the extreme situations but it's a bit of a fallacy to just train for these extreme events when in reality they are literally the tip of a very big iceberg of 'lesser' assaults.

Most of the time we are not going to be using deadly force and every situation will require its own unique level of physicality, or it might not require any at all.

Anyway, many of us can't reach that level of extreme violence from the off. Our go-to isn't to bite someone's nose off or gouge their eyes out. But we had better also prepare for those deep occasions too. And we will do that later in the book once we have learned everything else that is more likely to happen.

But here's the thing - you can usually, potentially, stop things from escalating and getting to the deep. And you can do this at every stage of a self defence situation, whether deep or early or in the middle somewhere.

Isn't that something you'd really like to learn?

CAN I REALLY BE STRONGER WITHOUT GOING TO THE GYM?

Another one of my big promises in this book is that I am going to make you stronger. I hope I manage to achieve all my big claims because otherwise I'm going to look the complete fool in front of all of you! So let's raise the stakes even more, eh?

Even if you're a trained martial artist or competitive fighter, I bet in Part Five there will be one facet at least that will increase your hitting power massively! Maybe even fifty to a hundred percent! That is how much I trust The Magic Five.

For the rest of you, making you stronger is not going to be difficult. I am telling you that by the end of Part Five you're going to be able to hit harder than you thought possible. And I must deliver that to you. Of course, this is a book and not quite the same as having me watch you and adjust what you're doing. But still I know what you can achieve with some practice.

So my main claim is that I can make you a lot stronger - more able to resist being pushed so easily or getting dragged. You will be able to push someone several times harder than you can right now, but this comes with the caveat that... wait for it... you must practice!

In fact, if you just did a few reps and followed some of the tactics shown you'll be stronger in so many ways. But just reading about these techniques and not practising them will be much less effective, as you know.

By the the end of Part Five you will be stronger physically, as in you will always be able to apply more forces from such things as leverage principles and biomechanics rather than just using muscular strength.

Did you notice that now I've said 'always' be able to apply more forces? Well, I did!

It doesn't matter how old you are or what your current fitness level is, or if you're skinny or not, you will be able to generate more force if you apply the principles in the book, and especially if you add any or all of The Magic Five.

So many claims and I don't even need to make them because you've already bought this book! If I fail then I'll just look silly. But you will learn certain principles that will enhance pretty much anything physical that you do from this day onwards.

Whether you're digging your neighbours garden when they're on holiday and you want to annoy them, or you're using a hammer to smash rocks in prison, or you're taking on a new sport, you will be physically more capable if you apply The Magic Five to your endeavours from now on.

Just one thing - I am not saying don't go to the gym anymore. In fact, the stronger and fitter you are, the greater your chances of beating a bigger/stronger man, right? You know that. I'm just saying learn these principles and you will always be able to enhance your current strength level, whatever it is at the time.

Having good strength, cardio and flexibility will help you to fight longer and harder, and to run away better. Good flexibility makes a huge difference in how you can slip out of holds or from underneath people and get to your feet to escape. So keep keeping fit.

Overall how you will increase your strength and cardio in here won't be by adding muscle, flexibility and endurance - though if you actually practiced the skills in here it will add to those - but you will increase strength using structures and frames, movement and techniques. Once you learn these things they can be applied to other parts of your life too and be with your forever.

Isn't that a great side effect from just reading a book?

THE TWO BIG RULES OF SELF DEFENCE

1. TRUST YOUR INSTINCTS

Use your instincts. Don't close them.

They saved your ancestors, your entire gene pool that's led all the way to beautiful you, and they'll also save you.

Trust them.

and

2. DO. WHAT. YOU. NEED. TO. DO.

To survive. Do whatever you have to do.

Trust your instincts and do what you need to.

Those are the first two rules of self defence.

Remember them.

PART TWO: UNDERSTANDING THE BAD GUY AND UNDERSTANDING YOURSELF

"If you know neither the enemy nor yourself,

you will succumb in every battle.

If you know yourself but not the enemy,

for every victory gained you will also suffer a defeat.

"If you know the enemy and know yourself,

you need not fear the result of a hundred battles.

Sun Tzu The Art of War

Chapter Three, Verse 18 - Attack by Strategem.

Sun Tzu was a great philosopher and general in the ancient Chinese army. I'll keep it as vague as that because you can search him online if you want to know more. I don't want to waste your time. But the book he penned, The Art of War, is still lauded by the top military ranks in the world today. It is essential reading for them, including British and U.S. generals and senior officers. The book is also adapted to business strategy by some of the top business people, and it is sometimes studied by martial artists as well as others. I've read and studied and contemplated it several times and can genuinely say it is pretty amazing. It is worth a read. I might just work through it one day then fully apply it to women's self defence - but that might take me a while since it's quite a profound book and requires deep contemplation, while sitting under a cherry blossom and listening to a stream. It's too rainy and cold most of the time in England so I can only do that for about three months of the year at most.

What Sun Tzu says in the above quote really does apply to you when it comes to self defence.

We really do need to get an understanding of our potential attacker and we need an understanding of ourselves too.

So we're going to do that throughout this book.

Even though he's Sun Tzu, he forgot to mention that it's a decent idea to also know the locations and situations you could face. Tut tut, Sun Tzu. You should have thought of that.

So we're also going to do that too, as we work in layer upon layer and build your ability to defend yourself.

These are the skills you've been looking for so let's start building them and and make them yours!

THE BAD GUY:
YOU ARE NOT FIGHTING A MONSTER!

We will be dealing with the Bad Guy as we go through this book but I wanted to start by saying something very important. That he is a man. He does not have the powers of a monster in the sense of all-powerfulness.

He is not an unknown entity, though that is how we often see him in our minds.

We can't see him as a monster. Monsters are scary, undefeatable and unknown. They scare us because we don't know what powers they have or what their weak points are but we do know those powers are most likely beyond our own and their weak points are few and far between.

Yet isn't the reality that once we know something about a monster we can usually beat it?

A snake is a scary thing for most of us. We don't want to really encounter one in any given situation - and I've encountered way too many on my family trips to Kashmir. Sometimes in the bathroom if you don't check before you go in, and often in the yard, where they slip under your charpoy cot to get some shade from the sun but you only notice them when you get your feet off the cot and start to slide them into your sandals. The thing is that even with that 'monster' lurking around everywhere, once you learn about it, once you know what it basically can and can't do, it basically becomes a game of strategy and tactics.

If you're going to the toilet, just stop at the periphery and make sure you scout around properly - including inside the bowl - before you fully venture in. If you're lying on the cot shading from the searing midday sun you better first just pop your head over and take a look underneath before you get your sandals on. And if you're heading out for a walk, you should always carry a big stick, and maybe a machete. You never know what's going to walk across your path. I've genuinely had a wild boar, a wolf, many snakes, large poisonous lizards and giant biting bullfrogs the size of watermelons that I can remember off the top of my head.

A snake is scary indeed, for me anyway, but I learned how to check for them and I also worked out how a long stick will take care of one that maybe scared me more than the others.

The same applies to any other animal or monster that scares us. They're monsters until we study them and figure out what they do. Then we can craft tactics and skills and equipment to beat them. We can train to beat them at a game where maybe they had the upper hand on us before - but now they won't.

So for self defence, it is a man we are dealing with. Truth is that morally he might be a monster and quite reprehensible right now but he exists in form like every one us. He has the same limbs and body we have. The same weaknesses as the rest of us. He moves in certain ways and with his gait and ranges of motion set by limitations. He distributes his weight in particular ways. He is not beyond the laws of biology or physics or chemistry that control him like they control every one of us. He cannot jump over mountains in one leap or break bricks on his temple as if he was hitting himself in the head with a cream and chocolate Eclair.

He too is aware of this fact that he is human, which is why generally he won't suddenly approach you and suddenly start to fight you. That can happen but it's not that often. In reality he is likely to observe you first and only make an approach when he thinks he has a very good chance of getting what he wants AND getting away with it. In other words he will have assessed you and assessed the location (probably earlier) and is continuing to assess the situation - are there witnesses, are the vehicles driving by etc.

Only then will he approach, when he feels he has the upper hand. Now, you might not see him until he gets close to you, but he will have made those assessments. He may have spent only seconds making them but he will have done gone through that process. (We're going to have tactics to deal with all this but just for now I want you to understand the situation).

As he approaches, he will continue assessing you and the situation that is unfolding all around. He will abandon his act if he believes he is going to struggle or if he is going to be caught.

Once he has approached, he will assess if he can bypass your natural instincts to protect yourself. He has to assess if he can get past your physical barriers too, if you have any. Then he will use trickery and deception and nice words to get past your barriers and will only strike if he believes he is totally safe to do so and there is a strong likelihood he can accomplish the task he has set himself.

If he thinks he won't accomplish his task or he thinks he might get caught, he is very likely to abandon his entire plan.

And that is exactly what we are going to work on in Part Three of this book. We are going to develop the skills to show him he doesn't have a chance. We are going to physically and psychologically block him and challenge him from the very start so he knows this is not going to be an easy day of work for him. We are not going to let him get us to places where he won't get spotted by witnesses.

And should he still try then we are going to be ready for that too.

So we are going to learn about this Bad Guy as we go along and learn his tactics and techniques and how to nullify them from the off.

We so have to understand though that we are working against a skilled person, one who has rehearsed this in their head at least, and most likely in real life. The person who does these things, especially robberies and sexual assaults, is often a recidivist, a career criminal. He's done this many times. He's got a lot of experience at it. That's not to say that an opportunist won't take their chances; they will - and these skills will work against them too. But the majority of times we are dealing with someone who has a criminal background and has progressed to this level over a lifetime. He has practised and honed his methodology.

He will often be a slippery snake and a master manipulator but not a physical monster.

Which brings us to that man who really is very strong and you're forced to deal with him.

The first thing is that we have so many tactics and techniques that prevent escalation at every stage. We don't want to be in a physical confrontation regardless of whether it's an average man or someone as strong as a scafffolder. We will do whatever we can to stay out of it. A very strong man can physically overpower you for a while though. In these rare cases, you will feel powerless for a duration but he can't overpower you for ever. (Please refer to the chapter titled Moments of Power to get insight into using this as a tactic).

Plus all the skills in this book work against the very strong man too. He might be very strong but he will be unskilled. Very few people are trained to fight and what you will learn here are skills tried and tested against fighting athletes; big and strong fighting athletes. But as a woman there could be on some occasions a great disparity between your strength and his. Most of the time though this is not the case. Most attacks on women are by 'average' men. They're rarely hulky and strong. But should this person be of more strength than usual then the tactics in this book will help you a lot.

Here's the truth though. There is an end-game. You can lose and you can even die while defending yourself. That's the reality of it. There can be check-mate. And that's another reason we don't want to stay and fight, if we can help it, like martial artists do. That's also why we want to deter and make the whole thing awkward so that the Bad Guy can't progress and just leaves. And you know what, you're going to later discover some quite dangerous techniques too, that can really hurt someone should the need arise for you to actually deploy them. So keep learning, but remember that these skills and tactics will prevent most of what can ever happen. It's just that I also want to cover those one-in-a-million events too, so you understand you have the capacity to deal with that and therefore have even greater confidence to go about living your daily life.

You are not fighting a monster, and even if it feels like that for a short while, and you feel like you're completely overwhelmed, there will be moments when he's not fully in control. At that time you will have some pretty dangerous skills to get yourself out. So let's move onto the two characters you are most likely to encounter: The master manipulator first and then the career criminal (recidivist).

BE AWARE OF
THE MASTER MANIPULATOR!

I have met many master manipulators in my time in the police. Some that are worthy of their own tv series. And it's not the fault of the women who were manipulated . They definitely made mistakes along the way, no doubt about that. But the fault lies with the manipulator. Here's the thing. The manipulator has pretty much done this their whole life. It's like they've got a degree, a masters and a PhD in it. And they'd achieved all that by their teenage years. Their life now is probably a professorship. They live this way.

You cannot expect to survive someone like that without a thorough understanding of them. They're the master but you're not even a student. You're a vulnerable toddler that's not even walking yet in their world. Would you blame a baby for being robbed? No. So you can't blame yourself.

I have been involved in many stories involving these people. One male who deserves a particular mention worked on the Edgware Road where he plied his trade for a solid few years. He was in and out of prison regularly and every single time he was out he somehow met a female in the streets around Edgware Road, or the Marylebone and Oxford Street area. Here he approached woman after woman. He would watch them as they came out of the swanky hotels, then follow them and befriended those that he could. He pestered many and eventually one would give in and pass her correct phone number to him. He would store that for later use, whilst he continued fishing for victims he could get something from much sooner. His victims tended to be middle class women in good job roles. He often picked them up from the lobby area where he hung out if the hotel staff hadn't spotted him and suggested he leave. He would also wait opposite some posh bars to entrap women heading back home after finishing work early on a Friday afternoon, after they'd gone in for a swift glass.

Listen to this, it wasn't like he was attractive or dressed well in the slightest. He actually stank. His breath, his clothes, his body. Those teeth that weren't missing were mostly stained black. I'm not slating people for their looks or choice of dental hygienists. I'm just describing this man because he wasn't Craig Daniels or Brad Pitt, yet he manipulated women all along the Edgware Road area to Bayswater, successfully working his magic.

If you ever saw this man you would be as surprised as much as I was at what he was 'achieving'. You would tell me no way was he going to trick any of those women nevermind the number that he had.

I transferred him from a prison to a police station once, so he could be charged with a crime we'd proved he'd committed a year previously and I found his bank account had over £100K in it. His only form of income was his female victims.

When I spoke to some of them - often attractive, always middle class, working women as I have already said.

- they literally told me they had no idea why they fell for him, whey they took him into their hotel rooms or why they bought him watches and lent him money that they knew he was never going to pay back.

I could not work this out either. I know that whenever I dealt with him it was always after a stint in prison, and so his hygiene maybe wasn't up to scratch, but if Shrek ever met him, Shrek would think he was a catwalk model.

The only answer I could come up with as to why these very intelligent women, with good jobs, would fall for him was that he was a lifelong master manipulator. He knew, through a lifetime of plying his trade, exactly what triggers to push so he could bypass all their defence mechanisms.

I've met many manipulators but no one else was on par with this man. I wish I could have studied him but he spent more time in prison than he did on the streets and he wasn't an easy man to catch anyway. The good thing was that he was not a violent man. I suppose that's a good thing.

Another great manipulator I'd like to mention was a heart surgeon I dealt with. He was meeting girls in a particular bar in Leicester Square where he was putting tablets into their drinks and then getting them back to his home. He would buy them drinks at the bar and use his genuine credentials to lower their barriers so they didn't pay attention and never spotted what he was doing. When they got to his home, usually drugged, he would continue the drugging process through the night. He kept pills hidden in many places where you, as a guest, would never be looking. For example he kept pills in the tray of his plant pot. He kept them inside books on his bookshelf. He kept pills in certain shoes on the rack. He kept them between the mattress and the bed frame. This meant that no matter where he was in his place he could quickly access the pills and put them in the woman's drink. His drink of choice was Moet and he always had a few bottles cooling in his fridge. When he was arrested it was discovered that he'd probably been doing this for a very very long time and getting away with it. The only reason we caught him was because one of the bar staff at the London bar.

had thought they had seen him spike a drink and then secretly called the police. They probably saved a lot of women with that action.

Another crime that I once reported was of a man who ambushed a lady in central London. It would be unfair for me to say the exact place as it could lead to the victim being identified which would be unnecessarily unkind and unprofessional of me. This man seriously sexually assaulted the lady and only started the manipulation after the event. Afterwards. He cried and begged for forgiveness and kept the woman there until she gave him her phone number because she "felt so sorry for him". They then dated for several months, during which time he cleared much of her bank account of money. She was an educated woman, with a good job. When she came to report the entire story, and of course I tried not to show my jaw hitting the floor, she told me his name was John Doe. It wasn't John Doe but I don't want to use the real name. She told me his first name, one of the most common names in the world and said she had never got round to working out his surname. She described an average man of average looks and build and he lived probably within a few miles, though she had never been to his home, and his name was John Doe and he'd taken most of her life savings. She was very embarrassed by the whole thing and was barely able to relay the events to me without pausing to shake her head at her own "stupidity".

So, why am I telling you all this? Is it even related to self defence?

I want to make sure that you understand you are often dealing with masters of manipulation. Demons of deception.

It's why I continuously refer to the bad guy throughout this book as Bad Guy. I don't want you to be manipulated by him so easily, like I've seen on way too many occasions. It takes just a moment for these people to manipulate people like you and me. A millisecond of trust and he's through our armour and then he's got us. I'm not being paranoid. This is what I've seen and reported many times.

They're the masters; we're not even students. Let's never forget that.

So stay on your metaphorical toes and remember it's not your fault if you do make a few mistakes along the way.

Another major manipulator you should be aware of is the one who uses physical tactics to get at you. Some Bad Guys, either soon or at some point during contact, will try overwhelming you with the threat of violence. With these threats he might be openly aggressive and verbal or he might be quite more subtle. It could be that he's not loud but says something scary much more quietly, in a whisper. In this case it's most likely because he believes he will be overheard and someone could come to your aid. If he whispers, it might be worth considering talking very loudly and making sure what you say is clear to any listener that you are not cooperating with this person and in distress. He has given you the signal to do this when he whispered his threat.

If he does become physical he might start with gently ushering you to where he wants you to go rather than fully forcing you. This could be for a few reasons. Firstly because anyone seeing him ushering you is less likely to be suspicious than if they saw him shoving or bundling you into a room or vehicle. Another reason why he might gently move you is so that you are a little confused and so your fight or flight isn't fully triggered. In this situation you might be just moved along and go with him because you're not quite sure if he is a threat. By the time you realise he is, you'll already be in his trap. And so gently moving you is a tactic that works to his benefit in several ways.

Again, in these circumstances it is often going to be better to disobey him as soon as you can and be loud. If he's gently ushering you it's because he thinks there are people who might see you and he doesn't want that to happen. And if you do let him continue, and you go along with him, you are going to a place which is less safe than where you are now. Remember that. It will give you reason not to go with him.

So if he's being quietly demanding, or is gently moving you somewhere, you need to disobey soon and move away and be loud. And he might just leave.

THE OTHER TYPE OF LOWLIFE

Firstly, I'm not going to apologise for the use or tagging of this person as a 'lowlife'. I do not do it for socioeconomic or political reasons. I do it so you understand this person and you don't give them an inch when they approach you. At this time they are a lowlife because that is how they are operating. In the police these people were called Scrotes. Career criminals, recidivists, who got all their money illicitly and used it quite quickly to satiate various desires - including drugs, alcohol, new trainers and TVs - they otherwise couldn't steal. They're opportunists usually, always on the lookout, who take their chance as they go through their daily life, which always includes plenty of crime and Scrotey behaviour. They're usually the low end of the economic scale, living on a council estate where everyone is wary of them and has to lock their doors and hold on to their wallets whenever they see this person who makes their lives a misery. The Scrote will take everything from your car or home or your pockets and your wrists. Not just your property but they'll take bites out of the food in your hands and throw the rest of it on the floor so you can't eat it.

They'll urinate in your cutlery drawer and over your dinner plates during a burglary. Why? Just because. It's become their nature.

The likelihood of meeting one of these Scrotes is reasonably low for most of us who don't live near to them but it does happen. There is a chance we cross paths as we leave a train station or get off a bus and they try to take our property, like what happened to me in Manchester Victoria train station recently, which I'll tell you about in a short while.

The main thing we need to understand about the Bad Guy, whatever guise he comes in, is that he usually approaches with guile and manipulation. He often uses charm and asks questions to bypass our barriers.

An important thing to note is that although I have separated each of these into characters or individuals, I have done that mostly to highlight specific traits and tactics so you might spot them more easily when they are being used against you. In reality the Bad Guy uses all these traits, it's just the extent will vary. One Bad Guy might favour verbal trickery as his main method and another might prefer to be physically intimidating. But that doesn't mean that the one who starts with verbal manipulation won't swiftly switch to physical aggression. He might do. Most of them will use a variety of approaches and tactics and so from the very start it is important to stay on our toes and don't let them past your instincts.

GET SCARED! GET REALLY SCARED!

Fear and adrenaline are great friends of ours!

The British strongman Eddie Hall desperately wanted to break the 500 kilo deadlift barrier that was said to be physiologically impossible. Scientists, doctors and sportspeople alike said a human was not capable of lifting that weight but Eddie wanted to do it. He went to see many people who he believed could help. They all said no. There was no way a human could lift that. The bones and ligaments and tendons of the human body would not tolerate that level of stress.

But Eddie is Eddie so he carried on trying to find this person who might also believe the impossible was possible and help him get there.

Eventually he found a scientist who still said it was impossible…BUT wait, there might be the smallest of chances if they could trigger his fight or flight response. He asked if Eddie had heard such stories as when mothers had lifted up the end of a car when their child was trapped below? Or when a mother would fight off a bear trying to take her baby away? There were videos online where people accomplished unbelievable feats when pumped full of adrenaline and with the need to do some superhuman task.

It wasn't possible to lift a 500kg deadlift, not really, said the scientist, but he was willing to try. Eddie isn't someone who gives up too easily, after all, at one point he was the strongest human in the entire world.

So they practiced and practised firing his fight or flight. Getting him pumped full of adrenaline. He learned how to trigger his fear switch, get the adrenaline flowing to maximal levels and then control the result for his purposes.

On 9th July 2016 Eddie Hall lined up to deadlift what no other human had done before. Everyone agreed this wasn't going to happen. People who knew maths and science and levers and biology better than Eddie told him it was not going to happen. Ever.

But they watched anyway.

Eddie had 500 kilos on a weight-lifting bar sitting on the floor in front of him. Moments before he had triggered his adrenaline again and again and again and again and then walked out to lift this bar.

And I'm sure you've guessed what actually happened.

Yes, he lifted that weight, for the required duration, to set that world record that no one, except Eddie, thought was possible.

And then he immediately passed out! Shook like a jellyfish in an earthquake first and then passed out.

That day, adrenaline was Eddie's superpower. And what releases adrenaline? Stress.

According to the philosopher-teacher Eckhart Tolle, stress is caused by the perception that our future is not about to be as good as we want it to be.

There are other definitions of stress but this explains what creates it. Our worry about a perceived outcome. The more life-affecting we perceive that outcome to be, the more stress we get from it.

Self defence situations by nature are pretty high on the scale of life-affecting. If the outcome isn't in our favour then it might be that we lose everything. So stress is going to hit us hard anyway so we'd better understand it and use it to our benefit rather than detriment, right?

Stress and adrenaline are part of the fight, flight and freeze survival mechanism you've probably heard of. They are part of fear.

When we get scared or stressed, adrenaline starts pumping through our bodies.

At its best, a quick burst or three of adrenaline can save our lives or help save the lives of loved ones. At its worst, when we have stress for a long period of time, dripping in and breaking our souls, it will chip at our minds and bodies until they turn to mush.

That's how powerful adrenaline is.

Essentially it is a life-saver. That is its primary role, though in modern society it doesn't always work that way and it can slowly kill us too.

But you're not here for a sociological study or to learn about the effects of stress on health. You just want to understand it for self defence.

The three states that adrenaline and fear elicit are fight, flight or freeze. Now, you've probably heard of these three and have some idea of what they are, but it's worth going over again in the context of what we are doing here. I have read and studied fear for a long time. I've thought about it for a long time. I've felt it many many times too.

The basic premise of fear is to get you to fully focus on something that is going to potentially harm you right now. It wants you to pay attention and come up with a solution.

Pay attention AND come up with a solution. Right now.

That's what being scared is telling you to do.

It's nighttime as you walk across the beautiful African savannah. A warm wind is blowing your hair so it floats like you're in a shampoo commercial. You're holding hands with your beloved and the moon is shining on his lush hair too. *Does he use Head & Shoulders? Or maybe it's L'Oreal coconut gloss?* you wonder.

And then you notice two eyes reflecting at you through the tall grass about ten metres away.

You'd better pay attention those beady eyes being barely reflected by the light from your torch. And you'd better come up with a solution promptly.

Instant fear pumps you full of adrenaline, which goes into your bloodstream and does a whole load of good things. Much of these we don't really need to know except to take note that the whole point of adrenaline is to make you superhuman, just like it did to Eddie Hall. It basically gives you immense strength and physical ability right at that moment for a short while.

Store that thought in your head because it's important.

Adrenalin comes in dumps. That doesn't sound pleasant but that's what it does. It has to make you take notice right away and to act right away. That's why fear dumps a load of adrenaline into your system.

The feelings you have when an adrenal dump occurs usually start with shock. Mentally you achieve full focus on the task at hand because it might be the last task you ever do. Sorry to be morbid but that's what it is doing. When Eddie Hall went for that lift he said he didn't hear the crowd and didn't think of anything except that bar he was lifting.

So you'll focus on those eyes in the grass like your life depends on it. Which it just might. You'd better figure out quickly if they belong to a frog or a snake or something else. And right now you've forgotten about holding hands with your beloved, you've forgotten about the beautiful moon and you've even forgotten you were in a shampoo commercial. All you know is those eyes.

And the adrenaline pumping through your body is making it ready so you can run like the proverbial wind or fight like a wild animal.

Your blood is being pumped around your body at such a speed that your arms and legs and whole body start to shiver from so much excess energy in there.

Primed to get those muscles lifting a car off a child if need be.

It's the heart that pumps that blood around. And it's certainly pumping right now! You'll feel it hitting your ribcage as though it's trying to get out. You might feel the pulse at your neck or temple or in your biceps working powerfully to keep that blood and energy moving.

Your breathing will be hard. You need to get that oxygen driven into the muscles.

And at this time of survival you won't want to contemplate all the reasons why Schopenhauer annoyed and therefore affected the writings of Nietzsche. Nor will you need to craft a delicately written email so you don't annoy your boss who's going through a 'sensitive' time in his life right now.

In fact you only need your brain to do 'survival' things. And *immediate* survival things at that.

So you find your brain shuts off all thoughts not related to immediately solving the threat in front of you. It's why you can't write a sympathetic email to your boss and you can't contemplate Nietzsche's *Man and Uberman*. All you can do is fight or flight. That's all your body wants you to do. Get out or fight for your life.

Your mouth dries up too and you can't speak properly. You won't be able to sing complex musical arias right now. On the plus side, you probably won't need to.

And you'll also feel sick. And need the bathroom. At the same time. That digested and undigested food you're carrying in your body is really no use to you now. If you run or fight you don't want to be carrying that extra weight. It's not like you can digest it in time to use as energy for this fight either. So you need to get rid of it right now. And your body will be telling you that in no uncertain terms.

The thing is that you may have to release these liquids into the world, which is considered a cowardly and shameful act although actually it's as natural as breathing. We've been doing it since the beginning of time. So don't feel ashamed if you do it. Be glad your body is behaving like it's supposed to be.

It may also be that you want to and are able to hold back these urges. But here's something interesting – robbers and recidivists, in general, will abandon their game if the victim vomits or wets/poops themselves. Robbers don't like to deal with that kind of thing. They often back off even when someone starts to retch.

But there is one particular type who is sometimes not put off by these things. The rapist - he can work his way through quite a lot of things the rest of us never would. This is anecdotal evidence but it is what I have observed many times. They don't always do it but they seem to have an ability to bypass vomit and other liquids to achieve their goal. They're a different breed but we all know that.

One more thing about adrenaline. It will give you tunnel vision and tunnel hearing. This means you won't hear or see like you normally do, and then later you will struggle to recall what was said or exactly what you saw or how it happened.

Again, this is natural. The purpose is to focus you on what is happening. You don't need to hear the sweet sound of serenading starlings in the rooftops right now. You don't need to see or admire the beautiful vistas of the urban skyline right now. Your eyes and ears must focus deeply on the survival task at hand and that is what they will do, whilst eliminating anything they think is useless for your survival right now.

So there are many things that you might consider to be unhelpful happening to you. But guess what?

You are now physically primed! You are a beast!

You can really run and really fight!

So this is what happens when you get scared. When your brain thinks you're in danger. When your body is going to save you at all costs. These are all great things and we must use them as an advantage.

The fear. The absolute shear fear. Our bodily reactions to it are designed to prime us to be at our physical best.

That's it.

Once we understand this, we are not scared of the effects of adrenaline and can actually be happy when they show up in a survival situation.

The shakes are warming you up! The blood is pumping you to the levels of a superhuman. And your eyes and ears and mind are pricked towards the danger, focusing on it deeply so you're ready for it.

We have covered Fight and Flight but there is one aspect we still need to deal with in regards to adrenaline. It is called 'Freeze'. It's when you can't do anything. It's when your brain is over-run, overwhelmed, blocked, frozen, useless.

A select few know how to overcome it and you will be one of those after the next chapter.

AND GET ANGRY

HOW TO GENERATE ANGER AND OVERCOME FREEZE

In a self defence situation, you are very likely to become scared at some stage if not right away. We've talked about that a little bit in the chapter before this one. But apart from priming you for running or fighting there is one other thing that can happen to you when adrenaline kicks it. That thing is called freeze. It is when you just don't know what to do. It is when your mind is stumped and confused due to reduced blood- flow there. (Remember I said you won't need to think much and your body is preparing you to run or fight?)

So if you freeze, if you find yourself needing to take action but unable to do so, remember this…

ANGER TRUMPS FREEZE!

This is probably something else you already know but never had a good think about.

That anger is more powerful than fear and freeze.

Ever been really angry and notice how you blocked everything out of your world, only focused on what your anger directed you towards? And you wanted to fight, didn't you? You wanted to take action. And no matter how scared you were, or what the consequences might be, you were going to take action.

Now, maybe you've never been in such a situation. Not everyone will have experienced things to such an extreme level. But just take it from someone who had anger issues as a child, that's how it is.

Notice how in that situation above you were ready to go and were not mentally or physically frozen at the time?

Anger is good. For self defence that it. Otherwise, it's probably not so good! But we are only dealing with self defence situations here. If you've got anger problems then watch the film Anger Management with Jack Nicholson. That might cheer you up.

Anger trumps fear and freeze.

Let's say that fear overtakes you when you find yourself in a threatening situation and you somehow forgot that fear and adrenaline are your friends. All you feel is overwhelming fear at the time, and you get the shakes, and you can't talk, and all those things happen to you and this overwhelming fear makes you freeze.

But if you get angry, really angry, you'll suddenly find you don't care about the fear. You'll be angry and now focused on how to beat the cause of your anger. You will not be frozen anymore.

So we can work with anger in self defence scenarios. It can give us increased motivation to get out, especially in the more dangerous situations. And if we don't know what to do and feel stumped, we can use it to focus on the person we need to get away from. Let him have it all.

Here's the thing, you can actually generate anger yourself and you can do it very quickly, which means we can actually use it as a tactic.

CAUTION ADVISED: I am going to show you how to generate anger next. It might be wise not to go through this exercise if you're feeling a little sensitive and don't need the stress. It's not a very nice exercies but it is effective. You could always come back to it another time.

So right now maybe have a think about what could make you angry at this person who it trying to harm you.

What is it that's making you angry?

Maybe it's the situation he's put you in. You were on your way home to a nice meal and now this? Is it the fact he might damage you? Your body? Your face?

He's going to harm you, is he? He's going to touch you and destroy a part of your life for a long time to come, is he?

What if he kills you? Who will you be leaving behind who will be very upset? A child/partner/parents? What state will they be in?

Maybe it's a cat or dog you have. Or anything that you would fight for. Your job you worked hard for. Your career. Even the possessions you fought had to get.

Find the things you don't want to lose. Things he could deprive you of. People he will be hurting by hurting you and layer that with how he could also harm you. Layer these things one on top of the other and increase anger that way. Think of as many reasons as you would get angry at the time of a possible assault. The more important the things are, the more effects they have on your life, the more powerful they will be to use to anger yourself.

You could also have fewer things and focus on them repetitively rather than many different things. Just keep these going round in circles in your head, getting more and more angry each time you think about them.

And now you have a very good idea of how anger is generated.

Professional fighters generate fear and then anger in exactly this way. They do this all the time. They start doing it way before they get into the ring. If you watch the so-called face-offs before big matches they go nose to nose and stare at each other like bulldogs that have been stung by wasps. They've done that to themselves, to get angry, so they're not scared of the other person, who is a dangerous person in their life right now and could hurt them in so many ways, taking away their livelihood and respect and prestige and even their life. So before the fight, they wind themselves up into a controlled frenzy, then square up to each other in the ring, before fighting to hurt and damage, often wanting to kill the other person during the fight.

That's how much they have trained themselves to hate that person and be angry at them, trying to take away food from their kids' mouths, and so on.

Right after the fight they usually hug and become friends. Battle-worn warriors. Two of a kind. Brothers in arms. But literally five seconds before that final bell they were still trying to cause the other person brain haemorrhage.

It's a manufactured situation. They could have walked away three weeks ago when the contracts were signed for them to fight. They actually didn't need to be here in this life and death situation. They could have got a job at Tesco's. Instead they worked all this anger into their body and mind so they could fight to the death.

At least to some degree they had a choice in the matter. But the person who we face is not going to play a fair game! We didn't ask for this game, we don't want to join in and we are probably trying to get away. They dragged us into it to hurt us and get something for themselves.

So if you can't walk away, and they put you in real fear for your life or limbs, then it might be time to get angry.

Don't Freeze.

Get really angry instead.

PERSISTENCE & REPETITION

Rhonda Rousey is a multiple Ultimate Fighting Champion, which is a cage-fighting/mixed martial arts tournament. She made almost all of her opponents submit with an armbar. They knew that's what she wanted

because that's how she always won. She chose to win like that and every competitor knew that's what she was going to do.

Yet she still succeeded at it. Every one of her competitors knew she was going to try for it, and being mixed martial artists themselves, they all knew about it. It's not like it was a surprise move that no one had ever seen before. It's one of the old martial arts fighting moves that they all practised and they all knew to practice a little extra before facing Rhonda.

So Rhonda would get into that cage and soon she'd be trying to get that armbar - proper name *juji gatame*, if you wanted to know.

And guess what? It failed. And it failed again and it failed again and again. The fight would continue and Rhonda would have another go with this move that her opponent expected. And again it would fail and again. But Rhonda did not give up. And she's pretty mean in that cage too! Quite ruthless. She'll break off your arm when she gets it, without hesitation. They all knew that.

She kept trying and trying until her opponent broke down. And she won eleven fights in a row like that - with a *juji gatame* armbar against women who knew all about it.

Another fighter, named Mirko CroCop, a Croatian police officer (hence his surname being CroCop) literally used one move to knock out many of his opponents - a right leg kick to the head. He was another fighter in those limited rules fighting arenas where almost anything goes. He went for that head-kick again and again and again. With his right leg. And he would miss. And miss again. And miss again. But eventually he would get it, right to the head, of another professional fighter at the top of his game, who knew what Mirko was going to do because that's how he got most of his opponents.

The point I am getting at is that sometimes you just have to keep going and going until you get what you want. In our case it is some kind of escape that we want. We want to get away from the Bad Guy.

The second point I wanted to make was that there are some skills that work. That really work. Mirko knew his right leg kick was going to work. Rhonda knew the armbar was going to work. Yes, they are both trained professionals and you are not, but in here, in this book, you have the best skills there are. These are the skills that work in self defence. Again and again. Today, tomorrow and for eternity. For your grandma, for you, your kids, and their kids' kids.

With Mirko and Rhonda their opponents knew what was coming and so it took them a while to get those techniques to work. But work they did. The techniques that you will learn here are not ones Bad Guy will be expecting. So they will work much better than CroCop and the Rowdy one's did.

But what if he knows these skills?
Well, he won't.
But what if he does?

Well, these are the same skills that are tried and tested every single day in the self defence worlds and the martial arts worlds. They work against people who practice them every day and know them. These are also some of the skills that cops use every day. These are proven time and time again.

The skills you are about to learn really do work but I wanted to make sure that you are persistent in your fight. Persistent in the use of these skills but even more persistent in yourself because it is that inner resilience, like Rhonda has and like Mirko has, combined with these skills that is going to see you through the toughest of battles.

The Bad Guy might be resilient too. He might not give up at your first offensive manoeuvre. He's probably done this before and got away with it.

But this time he's met you.

Be more resilient than he is. That's what I want you to be. That's what you want to be.

WANNA SCRAP?

Scramble and scrap.

That's the reality of self defence. There is rarely such a thing as a neat technique or wrist escape or any of that in reality. Although you have to learn one skill at a time to focus and make it yours, the reality is that you will do many things all at the same time in a live situation.

He grabs your wrist. At the same time as pulling your wrist and getting your balance, you also poke his eye, whilst simultaneously shouting for help. Then, before the poke is even finished, you're already kicking him in the groin, which you know might or might not work, so you don't stand on ceremony to admire what you did, but have already moved onto the next thing, which is dropping your bodyweight to stop him from dragging you away.

It is rare to ever apply a technique neatly or singularly without a follow up. Techniques work but under duress and pressure they are nothing like they were in training.

In training we have to break things down into smaller components and show them neatly so you can see how they work. You start off light and learn the move and then you start to apply it under progressively. As your training partner increases the pressure over the training sessions, now it will start to get more scrappy and more like real life. You'll now start to do many things simultaneously and you'll see that attempts fail and you must just keep trying. It's not only you that has to do this. You know that. You're not so special that your one attempt will work but even Rhonda failed! The Bad Guy will also be failing, but every time he fails, he is losing time and getting closer to leaving. Every time you fail, you've just made another attempt and you've stumped him a little more. Your failures are even victories in self defence! Add up your failures. They're closing in on victory.

So in reality every technique you try will have to be applied whilst fighting, whilst scrapping, whilst scrambling, whilst falling, whilst getting hit, and you could immediately be under the highest pressure, without any warning, and adrenaline kicking in and all the rest.

I just wanted you to be aware of this before we move into some of the greatest techniques there are. I want you to know that these really work but you better practice them and you'd better be ready to scrap should the poopy fan turn up and hit you in the face.

PART THREE:
THE STAGES
AND SITUATIONS OF
SELF DEFENCE

PLEASE READ THIS ONCE

Welcome to the actual physical skills section! You are about to learn a combination of mindset, strategy and physical skills. Our aim here is to cover the absolutely essential skills that women really need to know, and to encourage you to practice these right away if possible. If you do this you will start to develop practical self defence skills. Skills you can use this very day.

We are going to use the 'street' as our reference point, not because it is the most common location for incidents but because the skills required here are all transferable to the home and any of the other scenarios. This dramatically quickens our learning process rather than going through each individual scenario and situation. We will talk about the common or less common situations when we need to and a little more specifically later on but what what you learn here will be applicable everywhere.

So in this section, you will get a thorough understanding of the most important skills and tactics you will ever need.

This is a progressive learning (and practice). We start with the skills you need to know first and build on that as we go along, adding layer upon layer of ability. Now, you might be tempted to get to the more juicy bits right away but if this is your first time going through this book then please just go through it in order because that is the way to make maximum gains right now.

You also might get a little confused if you dip in and out of chapters right now without going through sequentially because you'll have missed information and developments that you then need to employ in the deeper techniques. So first time around, please read through (and did I also mention to practice as well?! Haha!)

Another point to mention here is that there will be repetition as we go along. I can't apologise for this as it's quite necessary to make sure you have a wholistic understanding of the situations of self defence. It is a very big topic and to break it down to this digestible size has been a great undertaking. Sometimes we will need to go back a little bit to then move forwards again just so you get the whole picture. I want to make sure that you deeply understand this important topic and that is the only way to do it, to reference things back and forth.

As you may appreciate, not every physical skill can be coached via a book but you' ll see that a lot can. Without pitching a sale too hard, we do have online courses where you can learn in a more interactive way as well as get access to the team to talk to us. Check out www. power- for- women. org/ onestepahead and www.power-for.women.org

There's more you could learn than is in this book but then you are starting to move into the realms of becoming a self defence expert. You don't really need to know, for example, how to break arms or how to strangle someone with your legs. These are fancy skills and can be used in certain situations but they do not have universal application and are the next layer along from the absolutely necessary skills that we cover here. We will be making bread and butter. I am able to teach and do more fancy martial arts techniques but what you have here is quite enough.

So inside this book you will learn about every skill that you will ever realistically need. Remember that those guys on the street are not trained guys. I've dealt with them a thousand times and I know their skill levels are quite pathetic overall. However, I am fully aware that I am a trained individual, that I am a man, of average size, maybe more than average strength, and even without training they wouldn't always pose as much hassle for me as they would for a female who is smaller and not as strong. But then that's why you have this book in your hand! To deal with that man! Let's set the balance in your favour.

Also, just one more reminder that the physical skills and all the situations here apply in any location. It doesn't matter where you are. These moves are universal. You can use the same move to Get Up if you've slipped and fallen to the floor or if someone has thrown you there or you were already on the floor to start with. And it doesn't matter if you're on the beach or on the shopping mall toilets or in an Airbnb bed you've hired. The same move applies across the board.

You can use The Fence at home or on the street or in a corridor or in a car park, in your home country or when abroad. It applies everywhere. So although I'm using the street as an example, do imagine yourself in some of the places that maybe concern you in your own life and then transfer these skills across to those locations. There's also nothing stopping you from taking this book with you when you go travelling. You can open it up, refresh your memory, practice the skills for half an hour anywhere in the world. As I have said, this is a reference book as well as a study book and the skills in here won't expire until men grow two heads and a third arm. (Which might be in the next three years if Elon Musk has anything to do with it).

SHOULD YOU RUN?

Women think they cannot run as fast as men. This may be true overall. Some women will be able to outrun a man and some won't.

The only way to find out if you can outrun an assailant is to run, right?

Also, here is a question for you? Just because you don't think you can outrun him overall, does that mean you shouldn't run? That you shouldn't try?

No!

It's your decision and your consideration at the time but for a start you might end up in a much safer location just because you ran a few steps. A location where you might be spotted much easier than the one he was trying to take you to.

You may have been noisy and made a commotion as you tried to flee and that would have been obvious to an onlooker that you were trying to flee. The noise might alert someone.

Also, as you run you might spot a safer location and make your way to it now or even a little later.

If it's possible to change locations (to a safer location of course) or even get a little closer to a safer location or get somewhere you are more likely to be seen or more likely to be heard SHOUTING, then it was worth the attempt to run.

And whilst you're running, he's not hurting you or doing what he wants to do and you're breaking down his will and you're making him waste time.

He might not even chase you!

You're too much effort! He wants it easy. He generally doesn't want to have a difficult time.

This is where we need to evict movies out of our heads. Only in movies does the bad guy play cat and mouse and torture his victims in complex ways. In real life it is very very unlikely, especially on the street. In a house or building it might be different and he might give chase. But again, you are buying time, you might have better opportunities to get help or shout out of a window or door at the new location you reach, even if it is only a few metres.

The Bad Guy wants easy access to what he wants. And then he wants to get away with it.

So, running is good, generally speaking. The only point I would make with it, is that when you do run, if the man chases you soon is close behind you, be aware of not giving up your back or being tackled to the floor. You do need to stay on your feet as much as you can. If you run and he is going to catch up then face him asap, preferably get The Fence and fight him off from there.

If he is already close you should always turn to face him because you'll have a better chance of survival than him getting you from behind.

Breaking free and running/walking away could be a possibility at any time during an altercation - from the very start and all the way to the deep fight. So I just wanted to make sure it had it's own little chapter before we dived into the fighting skills.

Flight is always an option you should be considering at all times.

But you knew that. I was just making sure you remembered it.

So we've done a bit about Flight and we've done a bit about Freeze.

Shall we get on with a bit of the Fight?

Self defence comes in five stages. You're going to learn the skills you need to navigate all these stages, from awareness of a potential situation, to being in the middle of an early altercation, all the way to the deep end, where you're locked in a room with someone who wants to harm you severely. You're going to be ready for all of it.

I can't wait to guide you through this!

STAGE ONE: AWARENESS AND AVOIDANCE

Stage One is the stage of awareness and avoidance.

What does that mean in normal language?

Basically we want to avoid any conflict where possible and to do that we have to have an awareness of several things.

We must be aware of our location. Who is there? Is the location well lit? Am I going to be safe? Where is there a safe place if something happens? Is there CCTV? Where are the nearest people who could help me?

We must be aware of what we are doing. Are we fiddling with a mobile phone or checking through our bag or purse, whilst being watched? Are we standing and walking confidently or do we look like we are so tired that a child could snatch everything off us and we wouldn't put up a fight?

And we must be aware of what we have access to for the purposes of alerting someone to come help ur or protecting ourselves. A mobile phone. A panic alarm. A very loud whistle.

Awareness and avoidance work in many ways but awareness can help you completely avoid a situation from escalating.

It can even prevent a situation from starting!

You have just walked onto the street, after exiting the train station let's say, and are heading home. You aren't being paranoid, but you're keeping your eyes open somewhat and are aware of what is happening in your surroundings. Before you take your phone out to start texting, you notice some man in the distance has looked at you and looked away.

The fact is that because you have seen him, you are now aware of him and your brain will work its magic and figure out if he's of a suspicious nature and if you should avoid him.

You will notice if he is out of place, if he is watching you or other women. Maybe he's generally just looking dodgy.

Having clocked the signs, and your brain telling you to be wary, you can take action.

There are many things you could do but you can only do them because you became aware of this man who set your brain ticking.

Some examples of what you might do…

You wait until he's gone. So you stay (or go back to) the safety of the station.

You could call someone who could walk home with you.

You could go home using a different route or method of travel. You could get a taxi.

If he starts to move towards you, you might choose to put your phone away if it was out, or move your handbag so it's not so obvious. In other words you are making it more difficult for him to snatch your

property and secondly you're freeing your hands so they can be used if you need to fend him off.

All of these actions could cause him to realise you're aware of him and he actually never does anything. Or at the very least you're taking action and are not always one step behind him. You're ready for him.

On this day, just by being aware you managed to avoid any altercation and got home without anything happening at all.

Because you were aware you are now having tea and biscuits at home.

Let's say there's a day you're not so aware.

You walk out of the station, mobile phone to your ear, fumbling in your purse to get the bank card, so you can rush to the supermarket , which closes in fifteen minutes . You're generally not paying any heed to your surroundings, because we all know we get caught up in life, and the trains are late and time is running out and we're not going to make it to the gym if we don't rush or not see friends on time.

In this case, the first time you will notice him is either when he is approaching you or you'll notice when he's already grabbed you.

Is that the situation you want to be in?

Awareness really does work in many ways and it's a huge tactic to employ . In the book *Dead or Alive* , Geoff Thompson interviews various lifelong criminals who have violence in their blood. One of the things they say again and again is that if they were clocked early they were very unlikely to continue with their actions. Their aim was to catch those who were unaware and they left those who spotted them.

Have a read of that again. I think it is a really important bit of criminal psychology that is revealed to us there. That they are looking for those who are not quite as alert as the others.

Now, in no way am I blaming the victim at all. The victim is never at fault in my opinion. The Bad Guy is always at fault. He knows what he's doing to you and knows that it is wrong. But I want to give you the best advice.

If there is a chance that we can avoid these horrible men just by clocking them, just by seeing them, isn't that knowledge worth 2kg of golden saffron?

So being aware is a great thing.

"But is there a way I can fit this into my daily life, Hafiz?" I hear you say!

Yes! There is!

One of the main tactics I used in the police, and I believe it saved my life and limb many times (and I still use it in today in civvy life) is the Three Second Rule.

Check it out next!

GOT THREE SECONDS
TO SAVE YOUR LIFE?

The Three-Second Rule.

So this is a tactic I used regularly in the police - pretty much all the time. I still use it today no matter where I am. Maybe I'm on holiday or anywhere unfamiliar or familiar: I automatically do this without even thinking about it. You probably do something like it too but aren't so conscious of doing it. Being conscious of it allows you to deploy it as a tactic rather that it happening at random. With practice, over a little time, you'll do it automatically and turn it into a tactic, without even having to think about it.

It's a fact the Three Second Rule saved me many times by stopping things from even starting or at the very least allowing me to prepare for what was about to happen.

This is it:

Basically, stop where you are, for about three seconds, and just absorb what is going on out there in the world you just entered.

That's it.

When you arrive somewhere, you basically stop and take three seconds to look around and let your brain see what is going on.

You can use it in the most common places where women are attacked. One of the most common places for being attacked is near the home, usually as the woman arrives there rather than when leaving. Some stats show that 7 out of 10 attacks occur either at, inside or very near the home. You should generally pay more attention when you arrive close to home. Use the Three Second Rule and scan around. And you know what, you often don't even need three seconds! You know your home and the surrounding area! A quick glance will let you smell if anything is out of place or some odd-bod is hanging about.

You know what, you can even use more than three seconds. Push it to five or even ten if that's what you need to do, to stop and observe for a little longer. And often just one second will do. You can even do it while you're walking along, especially if you're familiar with the location, such as your home. I know it's called the three-second rule but I had to give it a name. And it was sensible to call it three seconds as that's

about the right amount of time. But you decide. You might need another scan too. You gave it three seconds and spotted something that requires more attentions. Wait and let the situation sink in. Scan again before you decide what to do.

It is a very good rule to use when exiting a train station or getting off a bus or out of a car as these are the times when women get robbed the most.

So The Three Second Rule works in so many ways and in so many places. Have a think now of all the places where your brain is often triggered when you arrive or leave and start making it a part of what you do when you arrive at those places. Think about where there are safe places nearby too, where you could get to safety or find a person of authority who could help you. Make sure you know the name of the road and any permanent structures that would help you identify exactly where you are in these places that concern you at this time. It is not paranoia. It's just a sensible practice to adopt.

I'll give you some examples of when I used it in the police. When arriving at the location of a 999 emergency call, prior to getting out of the car, I would have a good look around before opening the doors. I would be lucky to get three seconds to do this but I would always have a one-second scout. Just scan the lay of the land, who was there as an obvious hindrance and who was there likely to help (authority figure such as an owner of a venue or a police colleague etc) and who there was an unknown threat at this time but I'd be keeping them in my periphery throughout.

Before entering buildings we had to go into I would have a good look about at the doorway and listen before going in. I often had to walk into random buildings I'd never even seen before, down a back street, where I didn't know how I'd get back out. Housing estates built as complex mazes and suchlike. By using The Three Second Rule continuously, I assessed every new area I went into.

One of my observances in the Three Second Rule was to check the locks of the venue I was going into. You won't believe how many different types of locks there are and I really didn't want to be locked inside a building with a madman and his rabid dog, so I sensibly added lock checking to my Three Second Rule before letting a door shut behind me.

I've used The Three Second Rule before intervening in fights. A brawl breaks out between two drunkards in a very busy pub in the back streets of central London. One player on the screen kicked the ball and it went too far to the left and that's enough reason for two opposing football supporters to start a riot usually, so I've found. So I'd pause for a second at the entrance and see ten of their mates running towards the altercation that I would have been in the middle of if I hadn't given it a second or two. Now I could deal with it from the outside heading in, rather than being inside it and have the ten guys surrounding me. It also meant I could call resources to the scene and save more people in the grander scheme than be stuck in the middle of a fight knocking out ten drunkards to save myself and them.

The Three Second Rule has many uses.

Make a habit of it. I know it has saved my life innumerous times and it will do the same for you.

Quick examples of where you maybe could use it:
Use The Three-Second Rule when arriving at or leaving your home.
Use it in the car park when you arrive at work, before getting out of your car. Use it when you leave your work building in the evening and you're alone. You can use it when getting off public transport on your way home.
You can use it when walking to the ladies room of a large but quiet restaurant or a club or a bar.

Think about it for yourself. Where are the places you might integrate it? Also learn it as general tactic that you could employ in any given situation. Imagine if they used this tactic in horror movies. The victim-to-be just stopped for three seconds and had a think about it before they went in somewhere. They would avoid all that hassle – but then there would be no more horror movies! So let's not let that happen because I like horror movies! No Three Second Rule for them.

But in our personal lives, The Three Second Rule might just help us avoid the monster many times. So maybe you should know it and apply it.

CALLING THE POLICE

So you're aware and you spotted this person. That doesn't mean he won't still approach you. It's just less likely he will, because you've clocked him and he knows you're on your toes.

One good thing is that by you being aware of him he is unable to ambush you. If he does approach it will be from the within sight. This means you are more likely to naturally turn towards him and face him and so now you are starting to reduce much of what he can do. You are also more ready to deal with him than if you were if he jumped on from behind, where you would be playing catch-up from the start.

If you've become aware of someone who's clocking you and he's still at a considerable distance rather than close by, you may have time to think about what you have on your person that could help you right now.

There's your mobile phone. Maybe you have time enough to call the police?

Here's the thing with calling 999 - they record the call every time.

So you don't need to have a conversation with them. You don't have to be polite and nice and introduce yourself and tell them the whole story.

You could just spit out your location and that you're in trouble.

Those are the two most important things they need to know to get them in action.

Your location. "Hello, I am at…"

And that you're in danger/trouble/need their help/are scared etc.

Be clear. Repeat it if you want to and if you can. But that's the first most important thing they need to hear. You should shout out the street name, if you know it, and the number of any door you are nearby. That makes your location very precise to them.

If that is all the information you can pass over before the call is cut they will send someone to that location.

In the U.K. if a call is cut off the police will investigate it as a priority and send someone there.

So, what if you don't know exactly where you are?

You could check the map on your phone if you have time and a data connection.

If that is not possible, the next best thing is to identify the nearest obvious landmark. This could be a restaurant or hotel or church or leisure centre or shop. Anything that is obvious.

Name the place. What is the name at the front of the restaurant or the church or the chippy? What else is there?

Of course the house number with a street name is going to be the most accurate way to say where you are. But you can name other obviously visible objects like a post box or phone box or even a vehicle/car. The type (a blue van, an SUV, a big red car, a small hatchback) or colour or make/model will do. Police are usually good with vehicle makes and suchlike.

If there is a hotel/restaurant/church or any social place there will be potentially helpful people in them. You should already be heading that way. Even a busy road is worth walking to because passing vehicles can be witnesses or they might stop or they might call the police.

So your location is the single most important thing to know when contacting the police.

Next, if you have time and the means, you can describe the Bad Guy, the 'suspect'.

Start by saying it's a man (or woman if it is a woman!).
Then a description of their body: average, fat or thin build will usually cover this. You are not making a commentary on their lifestyle or their dietary habits. You are simply providing a description that will help to spot this person right away when police arrive.

You can describe their perceived ethnicity: appears to be white, black. Asian, Chinese, Arab, Eastern European, Southern European (Greek, Italian, Spanish etc).

Again, you are not making any judgments, you are simply saying what is observable and allows them to be quickly identified when police arrive at the location.

You can give other descriptors too, such as height (very tall, average, very short), or distinctive items they've got (red baseball hat, blue coat 'Moncler' written on it, diamond earrings, white Adidas trainers, Gucci man- bag etc).

You will give these descriptors if you have time. More important than descriptors is what is happening and the severity of it. Note how I said the severity of what is happening so the operator at the other end of the phone is not left any guesswork as to the level of threat imposed at this time.

So, as an example, I would say something like this:

"I'm on Marylebone Road, I can't find a number but I'm in front of the eye hospital and there's a red postbox here. There's a man following me and he's screaming at me. I'm going to get attacked any moment…"

NOTE. It doesn't have to be in this order. If you forget and jumble it all up it doesn't matter. Just get out the info you can. The call is recorded and can be played back and listened to by the police. And if it cuts out you're likely to have people running to you directly anyway.

In a normal situation the operator will ask you questions and most likely keep you on the line until help arrives.

If you're calling the police (or anyone else).
LOCATION FIRST

What dangers/situation you are in

Suspect details (build, height, skin, basic clothing)

Who you are

IDENTIFYING A REAL
POLICE OFFICER

There has actually been a major problem throughout London with robbers pretending to be police officers but it hasn't really been picked up by the media.

In the Sussex Gardens and Paddington areas this is rife. Many tourists and other unawares are robbed by men who pretend to be undercover officers, flash their 'badges', then take watches and money from victims to "test if they are fake". This occurs in central London all the time.

Another thing you might be aware of is the recent dregs of actual policemen having been dug from the deep pits they'd been hiding in for a while. Some have turned out to be killers, others serial rapists and paedophiles. I even knew some of them, unfortunately. In these last few years there seems to be no end to them, being discovered one by one but it's only scratching the surface of a small but bad disease.

So there could be a need to identify a police officer for various reasons. Here's the thing, the sexism, racism, homophobia, beatings and bullying all seem to occur when cops are on-duty and in uniform, and usually with other cops.

The serious sexual assaults and murders tend to be when they are off duty, pretending to be working and usually operating alone.

Cops work in groups and alone all the time but if someone approaches saying that they are one you might have the need to verify this.

Again, this is not legal advice. It is not advice from the police. It is the exact same advice I give to my sisters.

The only way to find out if someone is a real police officer is to call the emergency number.

Call 999 or 112 or 911. These all work in the UK.

Tell the operator your location and what is happening right now (that you've been stopped by a police officer) and that you want to know if this is a real police officer doing their job right now.

Do this from your own phone and make sure you dial this yourself.

The operator will be able to figure out if this is a real police officer. They will be able to check if this person is on duty right now. Or not on duty. They will be able to see if the person is assigned to the area you are currently in or they are operating out of their area. They will be able to check what their current duties are - should they be in an office or should they be patrolling this exact location in uniform (or plain clothes) right now.

If there are any discrepancies, the operator can advise you or send someone to you. They might speak to the officer/person to get further clarification of who they are.

Doing this allows the control room to become alerted if something is out of place. And it lets them know where you are.

The fact is that when officers committed the more heinous crimes they were usually off-duty but carrying police equipment, so they looked legitimate. They also had access to their warrant cards (police badge/identification badge) and so came across as legitimate police officers – because they were! So it is important to identify them if you're concerned at all. The control room will immediately figure out that the officer is not on duty and wonder why he is doing police duties when he's not booked on.

This is the only safe way you can really check if someone is a real police officer and/or on duty right now.

An officer should not refuse you making these checks either. If they're refusing then that's something that should concern you.

So if you are in doubt when approached by an officer, the only real way of getting near the truth would be to call the emergency numbers.

There is currently talk of male officers not approaching women alone in London and only doing so in twos etcetera but it still applies that you can call up the emergency number and get verification that they are police officers and currently on duty as well as in the correct location for their current tour of duty.

Most police officers are not bad though. It's going to be rare that you come into contact with one who is out to harm you. Most will give their life to protect yours. But this issue of bad cops seems to be something that is understandably concerning women in the UK at present and I wanted to show how to verify an officer and stay safe should you need to.

SOMETHING ABOUT ROBBERS

Robbers are looking for an easy life. They want to engage quickly and get away quickly. They want your property and they don't want you. If they've snatched your bag then you need to let it go, get yourself to a safe place, then call the police. Going after them or fighting them off is not a good idea. You don't know who this person is and what they're capable of and how many accomplices they've got hiding round the corner or if they're carrying a weapon.

Your best bet is to remember where they went and where they came from. You should try to clock, or even better, quickly make a note of what they are wearing. These people often wear the same clothes for every robbery. I recall a nasty schoolboy robber in the Tooting area of London. He would rob schoolgirls, smacking them first without warning. But the thing was he always wore pink Nike trainers that nobody else ever wore. We never let on that his victims had always said they were robbed by a guy wearing pink Nikes and so we always knew it was him. It took him over a year to figure that out before he went for white and red Nikes. (I am not blaming Nike for the robberies. I believe the boy did these of his own accord). Now the victims told us they were robbed by a boy wearing white and red Nikes! I'm not even joking.

Robbers are usually ready to take the opportunity. They generally haven't planned nor pre-selected their target prior to them spotting one. They are looking for someone 'vulnerable 'at the time. Someone they

think isn't paying attention to their surroundings, and they will have watched the person fiddling with a phone, purse or something valuable they don't want them to have anymore.

They are most likely to approach you immediately, from your blind-side, and snatch the item and leave. They are less likely to come at you face on and demand the item, thought that does happen frequently too.

They often snatch the item and pass it to a friend who then walks off with it while the initial robber blocks your path and threatens you with their physique.

Another way to get robbed is by someone on a bike. This is also quite a common tactic. These people will be cycling very close to the pavement or actually on it, and they will be paying attention to people on the pavement rather than paying attention to the road like a non-robbing cyclist would do. They will snatch and bolt quickly on the bike. The best way to avoid a bike-robber after spotting one is to move away from them (with your back against a wall) whilst putting your phone and bag out of their reach. They usually rob while in transit and if they can't reach your items it reduces the chances of them grabbing anything.

The so-called 'hugger-mugger' is another technique I've seen hundreds of times in the Soho area of London and other busy party areas. I've seen it used effectively by individual robbers and robbers working in gangs.

What happens here is the 'friendly' robber will approach, all smiles and happiness, and put an arm around your shoulders or waist. As they do this, they or their friends will search your pockets and dip into your bag whilst you're trying to peal off the initial over-friendly cuddle you didn't ask for.

The key thing for your personal safety is to not let these people overwhelm you. If you haven't immediately shaken the 'hugger-mugger' away (because you're too polite or whatever and you've got a couple of drinks in you) he will continue hugging you and walking whilst he and/or his associates take your property. You also need to be careful where he/they are leading you. I've often written reports where someone suddenly found themselves wandering around the back streets of Soho alone with four, five, six guys who had now become quite unfriendly and demanding. So it's always best to only move to places where there is more safety and more chance of being spotted and helped.

Personally, I am immediately wary of anyone who tries to put their arm around me in the street on a night out, but I wasn't quite so concerned about this until I saw so many robberies take place like this. I didn't know anything about them!

In all these scenarios you really need to start considering the use of The Fence to create a protective barrier around you, as this will prevent someone from pulling or pushing you where you don't want to go. (The Fence coming up soon).

STAGE TWO: THE APPROACH, THE ASSESSMENT AND THE PRE-FIGHT STAGE

So now the Bad Guy is approaching you (coming towards you but still at a distance) or has already approached (is near you).

If he is still approaching then for him to be able to do anything he needs to be within 'grabbing' distance. Only then can he take something or hit you or grab you. We have to be able to prevent him from doing those things and we have a strategy coming up in a minute for that. But we need to talk about this so we get an understanding of the situation.

Of course it might be that you scanned the area but didn't notice him and he suddenly appeared, right there, within reach. You didn't see him approach because he is sly and practised at this and he's good at it. Or it could be he was hiding.

The third thing that could happen is that you are ambushed and find yourself deep in the middle of a fight. We will cover that a little later.

So, at this stage the person is either:

approaching you.
has already approached and is starting a conversation.

We can also call this the pre-fight stage - things haven't kicked off but they could do very rapidly.

But if they don't kick off immediately the primary thing he will do is conduct an assessment. He will start a conversation and the point of that is to see if he can get past your barriers, using feigned kindness or threats.

He could also assess you and decide you're too much bother or don't have what he wants and so he walks away.

Let me tell you something that happened to me recently in Manchester Victoria train station as I was on my way to the airport. This will highlight some of what we are talking about.

So, to start with I'm kind of medium to large sized. I'm not scrawny. I'm not (too) fat. I'm not short either and I do appear to have some muscle. No way do I think I look like a target for anyone, yet here I was in a situation where I had to be on my toes against, no doubt, a hardened and highly experienced criminal.

The robber was a scrawny-looking guy, half my size and few inches shorter. I was heading up the stairs of the bridge with my phone in hand, staring at the screen trying to figure out if it was going to be quicker to walk to the next train station along (Piccadilly) to catch a train there or wait for my scheduled train that was currently delayed. So I was engrossed in the maps to get directions, to see how long it would take me to walk to Piccadilly and at the same time I was trying to keep an eye on an app that showed live trains and how they were running.

About halfway up the stairs, this scrawny character ran right up to me and said, "You've been taking photos of my mum. Show me your phone."

He wasn't what you'd call outright aggressive, he was more passive aggressive than anything. Pushy attitude. He stood a couple of steps ahead on the stairs and so was towering over me.

It was at this time that I realised I had my phone out, in my hand, and I had been walking around without a care in the world. After all, the station was chock full of globetrotters who would be witnesses, and I seriously don't see myself as someone you'd want to approach and fight (although I've been wrong about that a few other times too, but it's usually people who had the bravery of beer in them). And it was daylight right then!

My phone was in my right hand and I automatically put it away in my trouser pocket. Now, looking back at this, I put it away because I thought it was going to get physical due to how quickly he'd approached and I wanted my hands to be free to deal with him. I didn't actually hear what he'd said until he repeated it. "Give me your phone. I'm going to delete those photos of my mum you took."

It was then I realised what he was after and luckily I'd already put my phone away. If I hadn't put it away then the situation could have been different. He might have gone to snatch it. If he had friends he might have attacked me because he had backing.

I realised what was going on so I immediately started paying attention to the whole environment. I was a police officer in London for a long time but I also grew up in areas that required good vigilance to survive. So I glanced around but without taking my eyes off him. I wanted to see where his friends were because he obviously wasn't so brave or stupid to approach me on his own. But I didn't eye any friends anywhere.

At the same time as checking around (glancing but never taking my eyes off him), I was fully aware of his body language and watching his movements, in case he took a shot. Something I should have done here is created some kind of Fence (coming up in the next chapter) so this was a big mistake of mine and could have meant I was a step behind rather than a step ahead and ready. But I also have a lot of fighting experience and have a fighter's sixth sense for knowing when someone is about to do something. People have hit me or tried to hit me in the tens of thousands of times, in training especially, so this is ingrained into my body (I think).

I told him that I hadn't taken any photos. Which was true.

He laughed. Then he started mocking me by making sounds similar to what I had just said. Mimicking me, parroting me to make fun of me. And as I thought about that, or my brain automatically considered what he was doing because it was extra-ordinary and not normal, he did a tiny movement forwards to check if I was ready for him if he hit me. He kind of flicked his body forwards. He was checking to see if he could hit me.

I was ready and also just out of range. Decades of training and practice.

But he did it twice again, immediately once after the other.

Now it had become a tactic to scare me. Checking if I'd stand up to him or if I'd capitulate.

I didn't move because he wasn't going to reach me easily from where he stood.

He did this a couple more times, pretended to come at me in what would be movements so small you'd only notice if you were where I was. Any passer by probably wouldn't have noticed what he was doing. He continued mocking me too.

At around this time I was going to back away, move off whilst making sure I couldn't be attacked as I did so. But he turned to walk away first.

At least that's what he made me think he was going to do so I automatically relaxed, that this thing was over.

I actually let out a sigh of relief (I must have been holding my breath, which I hadn't noticed) and dropped my guard mentally, started to move away... when he turned back for a second attempt.

He had taken half a step away when pretending to walk off and now he lunged at me.

Luckily, I collected myself rapidly otherwise we would have been in a physical altercation. I realised this was a continuation of his testing me. He was checking my reactions; checking if he'd broken me; checking if he could take his chance.

But it was clear I was ready for him, and definitely not scared nor psychologically affected by his trickery and manipulation, and I was still out of reach at this time. If he had come within distance, where he could hit me, I'm pretty sure there was only going to be one winner. Those who know me well or have trained with me will be agreeing with this right now.

He repeated this a couple of times, pretending to walk away but suddenly turning and lunging towards me as if he would attack. He continued a mocking laugh that I can't describe in writing. He was just having fun now, playing with my emotions. He'd turned it into a game. Just enjoying himself at my expense.

He'd played this game many times before and was really good at it. He would have also have often managed to gain property in the process of playing his game.

And then he just walked off, with a gleaming smug smile on his face, as if he'd just done something he should be so proud of.

Me? I was quite annoyed about it. He'd played with my emotions, sent me up and down, and also put me under physical threat, just because it's what he wanted to do. I reported it to the security staff at the station but the Bad Guy had left by then and since no robbery had occurred there was nothing they could do. The robber had played a good game. I was definitely on my back foot for most of it though luckily I've got some good backup that he wasn't aware of and it would have quickly taken me to my front foot and him down to the bottom of the stairs, head first.

This incident was quite interesting as it covered so much of what an attacker would do. As you may have noticed, the contact might be verbal, with physical cues added to it and it can be mentally challenging and distracting. It can be scary too. In this instance he was also checking my physical responses by moving quickly towards me in a manner that's not so easy to describe in writing but was obvious to me at the time that he was testing me. He was testing me in all these ways all at once. Masterfully, I might say, if I was one of his kind, which I will never be.

I believe he would have hit me if he had backup and/or especially if I still had the phone in my hand. I have little doubt about that.

One other very important behaviour to note is that he kept looking around. Instead of looking at me and engaging fully, he would glance about every so often, all around him in every direction, even looking over his shoulder behind him several times.

This it is a very common and sure sign that he was about to do something. It is usually done to check for witnesses, in case anyone is watching. It is something men do in fights, such as during road rage, because they're about to do something they don't want witnessed. They glance around and check the area is clear of witnesses and then they attack before running/driving away.

If anyone is doing this, not paying full attention to you but looking around like this, they are very likely to attack imminently.

I'm going to say it again but in a slightly different way. If the person looks about, especially over their shoulders to check behind them - they look one side and then the other, quickly - you are about to get hit or your property taken or both. So, you need to act before that happens (move out of distance, hit him before he hits you, shout etc. Do what you have to do).

Please, listen to your instincts.

Going back to the conversation the Bad Guy might have with you, it can be a complex spider's web, and he's the spider, not you.

Do not fall for his tricks - there will be many of them. Do not get entangled in his web. Do not even engage. Be brief. Gently, casually where possible, keep moving away.

Move away quickly if you can do so. Step away to create distance. Find a reason to do so if that suits you better but the less information you give him the less he can bring back into the conversation to keep you engaged.

Start moving into one of The Fence positions,

Just to let you know, although in the above example on my way to the airport I failed to create a Fence, I have on hundreds of other occasions used The Fence, by moving away casually while still talking.

So back all the way to what we were talking about before I so rudely interrupted with my story. The point of this Stage (the approach) for the Bad Guy is to get close to you, assess you and then progress from there. This could include ushering you to a more suitable location (that he will already have scouted) or grab your property but it could also be that he walks away after discovering you're not going to be the easy target he was hoping for.

So if you are already walking and someone comes beside you and walks with you, do be aware of where you are heading.

Are you walking to a quieter location? Are you moving towards his vehicle? Where are you walking to?

Hopefully it's towards a safer location, or a place with more friendly people who will help you, or where you will be spotted more easily.

If he is still approaching and hasn't got to you yet, you may have time to prepare. To put your phone or wallet away. To move your bag to a safer place. There might be time for you to move to a safer location - under CCTV or closer to where you might be more easily spotted because there's more people walking by.

It could be that you were standing next to a canal or at the side of a road and now you can move so that you are in a safer place, and he is going to be at the more dangerous side once he gets to you. And if things kick off he needs to worry about swimming in Weil's disease and not you.

When I was on the stairs at the Manchester train station, he was higher up than me and so I immediately stepped back with one foot, so that way one foot was higher than the other on the stairs and I had much better stability to fight from. If I'd stayed standing squarely on one step, he could easily have pushed me and I'd have had to get my balance before I could fight back. By having one foot forward and one back (like in The Fence) I was not 'one step behind', I had far more ability to resist any attack, and also to deliver my own shots back at him if anything happened.

So guess what's next?

Yes - The Fence!!

In the grand scheme of things, this is one of the most important positions there is, and you're about to own it for yourself. Get on your feet and start dancin'!

THE FENCE

Every martial art has a starting structure. For example, you've seen the karate stance, or you've seen the boxer in his stance. All sports have a stance too. You can call it the starting position from where all things are done.

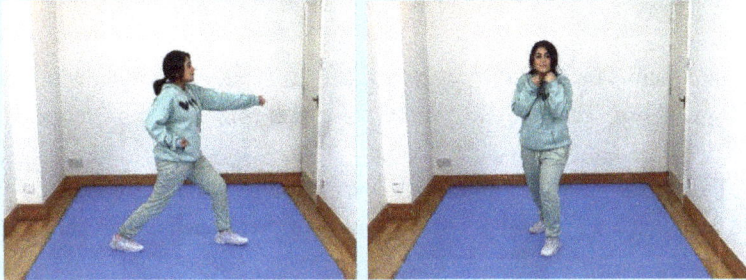

Above are the karate and boxing stances you may have seen before.

In tennis it's like this.

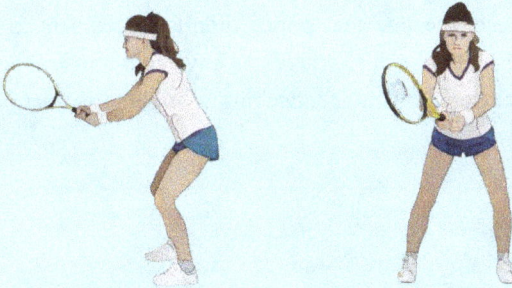

This is where the player starts from and this is the shape s/he keeps returning to again and again.

One of the jobs of her opponent is to make her break this structure, not allow her to get back into it often because that is how you damage her gameplay, how to make her make mistakes and start to fail.

In the police we had two stances. One was an obvious one, you've seen that one for riots, with batons raised and at the ready. Obvious to the observer/Bad Guy it's saying police are ready to go physical, so back off.

But there was also a stance that was not so obvious, that was not threatening to people. A covert stance. One that wouldn't trigger unnecessary physical conflict.

In policing, on the street, everyone is considered either a known threat or an unknown threat. That's it. Note how you always consider people a threat.

You either know what threats they wield, or you don't. If someone has a knife, you know what that threat is. If someone puts their fists up, you know what that means.

But you also have unknown threats. You might not know they want to punch you until they do. You might not know they have a knife and they're going to stab you until they do.

So you always have to consider people as having known and unknown threats as that was the best way to stay on your toes and stay alive. Policing can be a dangerous and pressured business, in case you didn't know.

The covert stance, the one that police didn't want others to see and feel threatened by was usually like this, where you have your arm crossed at about the chest, and the other one at the chin, scratching or rubbing or just pondering like Rodin's Thinker statue …

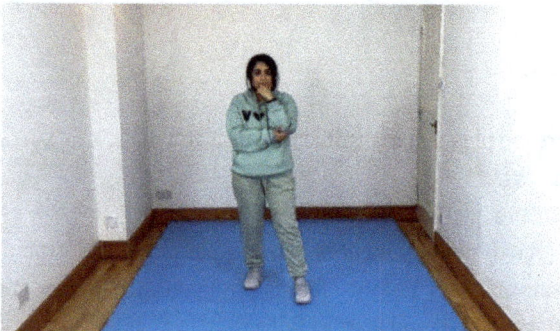

Or it was like this, where you're just rubbing your hands together like it's another cold and rainy day in England. Luckily, it's always a cold and rainy day, eh? Well, for 11.5 months of the year anyway, so this didn't look too odd.

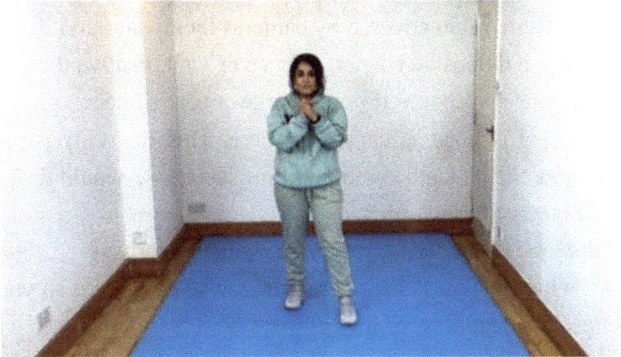

I bet you will now notice cops standing in these poses more often and you'll know why they're doing it! To have a Covert Fence, a level of protection and readiness.

So the police had a covert/hidden stance and an overt/obvious stance to deal with two different potentially threatening situations.

So what is the point of a stance?

The point is exactly the same as it is for all sports that use a stance, which is most sports. To be ready to act or react to anything that is about to happen.

To be ready to move position quickly as needed.

You are ready and focused on what is about to happen and you're going to deal with it. You are in a structure where you are strong enough to do deliver the forces you need to deliver, and resist forces that you need to resist.

So a stance, a structure of some kind, is SUPER IMPORTANT. If it wasn't then it wouldn't be employed in so many sports and in every fighting art there is in the world.

I know a very clever man, called Geoff Thompson. He created a few different self defence stances and even gave the idea a name: he called it "The Fence".

He actually created quite a few different stances for various situations but most of them only apply to men's self defence.

For women's self defence we only need two - one Covert/hidden Fence and one Overt/obvious Fence.

So The Fence is like a protective shield around you. Same as the fence around your house. Or the walls that make up your house and protect your property inside. These fences/walls are often covered by cameras these days and in a similar way we will also create a defensive barrier, a fence or wall, that we then monitor, just like you would your own home if you were aware of someone prowling around the perimeters. That is what is happening here. This Bad Guy is prowling. He wants to get at you. So we have to monitor him, just as we would the snoop who's lurking outside our house or garden.

So what does the Covert and Overt Fence look like for you?

Let's start with the Covert Fence and get you standing in it so you can feel it and get a better understanding of it.

You can, and should, use the the two Covert Fences that are shown above, that the police use, but there are a couple more that you might find more suitable personally.

This is one way you can stand in the Covert Fence.

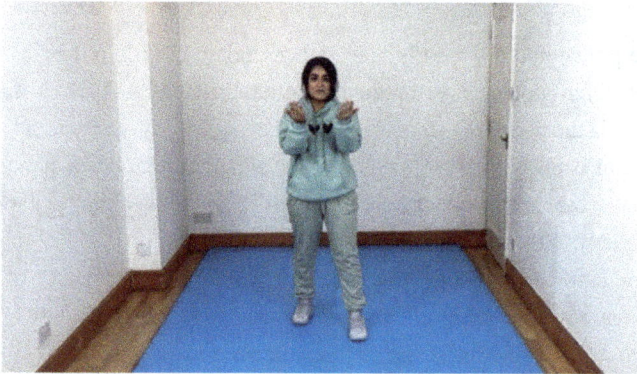

In this one you appear to be posing a question.

In all of the Fence positions your hands are raised and more able to deal with anyone coming at you, who might try to grab you or hit you. So always get your hands up.

You can easily push from here and run away.

You can hit from here too.

You are also far more stable on your feet than if you stood square and had both your arms down, and so the chances of you being pushed or pulled are reduced, or at least you're ready to act immediately if that should happen.

In reality, because you are being covert/discrete you'll need to find an excuse to put your hands up to chest/neck height, which is why the questioning fence works well, as do the chin scratch and also the warming hands. You've got excuses to put your hands up and you're not going to alert Bad Guy nor give him a reason to engage with you. An Overt Fence doesn't work in the same way, as you will see in a moment.

My go-to Fence tends to be as if I'm checking my watch for the time. I often lift up both hands as if I'm going to check the time on my wrist. And guess what? I don't even wear a watch!

You could also do it as if you're lifting up your handbag to check it or the contents.

If I have my phone in my hand and someone approaches me quickly I also lift up my phone to this height and pretend to be checking the screen but this could also work against you if you're about to face a robbery.

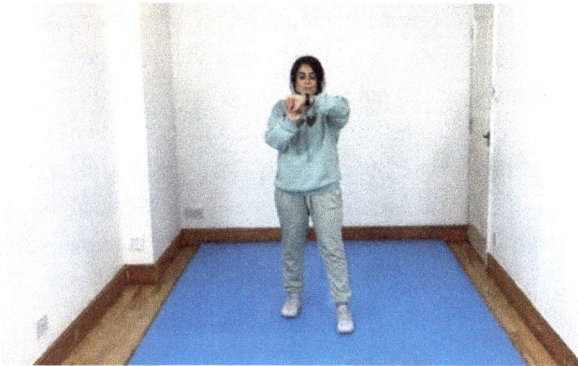

Any excuse will do. Find your own versions if you want, but get your hands up high. Having them low just puts you a step behind if he goes to hit you or grab you or push you. Your hands need to be up and ready. Whatever excuse you're going to use, decide it now and practice it so you don't stumble and have to think about it on the day.

The Fence requires you to have one leg in front and one behind, so you are able to resist pushing and pulling forces better. To do this without making it obvious requires a little skill. But you can just casually move one foot back a little bit when you start talking. He won't notice.

The way the brain works, by stepping forwards you're being a threat and therefore challenging him. We don't want to do that with the Covert Fence. In the incident that happened to me in Manchester, I stepped back one step on the stairs to keep stability.

Apart from the ability to resist his pulling or pushing, it also gives you the ability to push and hit harder from here.

But be ready. The Fence is a 'ready' position. Ready to take action.

Your physique needs to be strong. It needs to be ready to go. You need to be ready to act.

The Fence is a physical position but it requires mental engagement on your part. You are active in your eyes and head all the time, even when you don't appear to be to him.

The Fence also works as a psychological deterrent because you're not so easy to just grab as you would be with your hands down. You're not so easy to hit compared to when you had your hands down. It gives the Bad Guy something more to think about than he originally thought when he was approaching.

I have actually used a variation of The Fence twice with guys who were 100% intent on hitting me but they did not find a gap suitable enough to get through and so they didn't do it. These were 'men's' self defence situations and the Fence I used was not one of those above but tactically it was exactly the same. I used it to do the same things I've said above. It really does work magic all on its own.

So you know what the shape of the Covert Fence is but how would you use it practically?

I just want to make sure you are able to deploy it.

So the Bad Guy approaches you (or is already within grabbing distance). You should be in one of the two Fences. Let's say that he's approached and you don't have reason to use the Overt fence. He's not been aggressive and you don't want to trigger him or give him a reason to speak/engage with you. Putting your arms up into an obvious fighting stance (which is what the Overt Fence is) might give him more reason to stay and engage with you in conversation or might even trigger his ego into taking you on physically. So I tend to say to avoid the Overt Fence to start with and use the Covert Fence.

The Covert Fence allows you to create a barrier around yourself and gets you into a ready position to deal with anything that he throws at you but without him knowing that's what you're doing.

But what if he lunges at you, or touches you, invades your personal space, tries to grab you or hit you?

You deal with it (shove him off, hit him, whatever else you have to do) and from there you move into the Overt/obvious Fence.

The Overt Fence is your fighting position. This is the structure you will use and maintain if a confrontation turns physical. It shows that you know what you're doing. It shows that you are going to fight back.

Equally as importantly it is actually the best stance to fight from as well. You are ready to move backwards, forwards or sideways effectively. You are ready to hit effectively. You are ready to resist being pushed or pulled. It allows you to use your body to generate strong forces in every direction.

So have a go at it out now.

Whilst standing, put one foot back. This will be your right foot that goes back if you are right handed, and your left foot if you are left handed (about one in ten of all women are naturally left handed).

But do whatever is most comfortable for you right now. You can always change it later on after a bit of practice. Remember that you will be pushing from here, hitting from here, moving from here, and so to discover what is the right stance will be something you develop rather than figure out on your first attempt. You will get a chance to work more at this as we go through the book but right now have a go and get comfortable.

Consider if your arms would be ready to stop him moving at you or ready to shake him off if he were to grab you. Are your legs in position to be able to move about easily (so you might need to press down with your toes more than your heels, which allows you faster movement)? And are you able to hit from here should you need to?

You need to consider this. The Fence is a mental position as well as a physical one. Thinking these things systematically now allows you to have your limbs and body in the right place, and also to have your mind ready to take action. It will also connect your mind to your limbs right now.

Your hands should be about neck level. They shouldn't be higher than that and not lower either but about there, ready to fight. Of course, if things kick off, you do what you have to do, then get back into this position, including moving your hands back to this ready position.

Bend your legs a little so they are springy and ready to be used when you move or hit.

This is what the Overt Fence should look like.

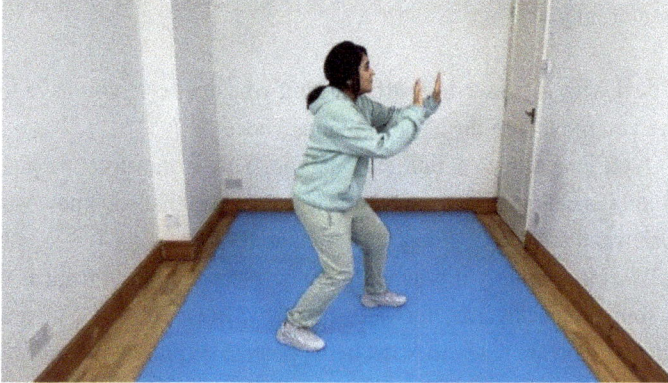

Your hands should not be pushed out all the way and shouldn't be pulled into your chest either. Somewhere in the middle allows you to resist forces if he charges at you but also to generate forces when you want to hit or push him.

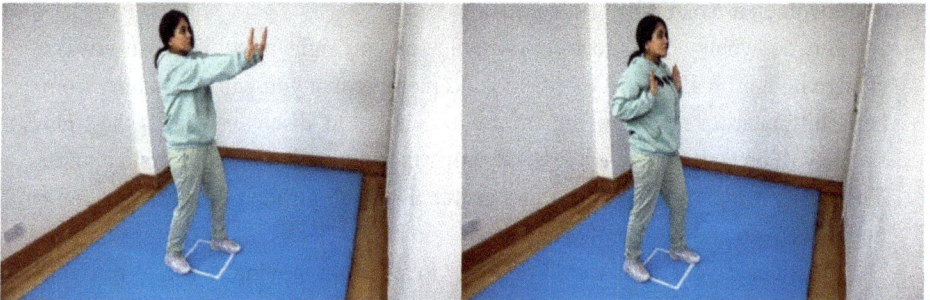

Whichever Fence you use (Covert or Overt), it needs to be mobile and ready to go. It is not a stiff structure all the time, like a building. It is a relaxed and mobile structure that can turn solid one second then be freely moving the next.

The Overt Fence tells him you know what you're doing.

I've seen it used by female police officers against men who were about to attack them and it stopped the attacker in his tracks. He didn't attack. Literally stopped moving forwards. Now, that was in policing situations so there are some differences to when you use it for self defence. But I just wanted you to know that it is a really useful tool and in itself could stop the attack from progressing. That's how good it is.

Furthermore, if any passer-by sees you in an Overt Fence, even from a distance, they will have no doubts about what you are doing - that you are fending this man off. It's obvious.

So if you've got reason to go into the Overt Fence (he's tried to lunge at you, or hit you, or touch you, or grab you for example, or you feel things could kick off any second) then get right into it. You might need to push him or hit him before you get into the Overt Fence. You might want to take a step back and get distance from him as you put it up. You might want to shout as you do it.

Practice these things from the Overt and the Covert Fence right now.

Always be loud too. There is rarely a time you should be quiet in self defence. Loud, vocal, and keep it that way.

The Overt Fence is a good time to start shouting at the person if you haven't already. A good thing to shout is

"GET BACK"
or
"GO AWAY"

You can shout anything you want but I have seen both of these work in live scenarios. I think the reasons are that firstly it is a command to the person (you're telling him what to do, giving him orders, forcefully) and secondly Bad Guy knows anyone within hearing range will be alerted and have no doubt you're in distress and maybe come to your aid or call the police. Shouting at him, injecting your words deep into his brain, can also have a psychological effect on him. So aim to shout loud so people can hear you far but also inject those words into his head with venom.

As I've already mentioned, you should take a step/s away from him when you get into the Overt Fence. I do that in the Covert too. I casually find reasons to just step back and then another step while I talk. I want to create more distance between us so he can't just grab me or hit me. I want to be out of reach to buy myself more time to react. Also, from his point of view, he is less likely to attack if I am out of reach as he can't do it with just one swift move.

So shout loud, injecting the words into his brain with venom, and move away whilst in your stance. Keep shouting for him to GET BACK (or use your own commands that you should decide on right now) and hopefully he will see you're not an easy target and just get lost. If he doesn't then we will need to fight him off and there's no better self defence stance than The Fence to start doing that.

So The Fence is a seriously useful tool in so many ways. We will work on it again and take it several levels higher, but for now, please just have a go at it and get comfortable with the shape of it. Understand the structure and the reason why your arms are up or why you're standing in the shape that you are.

As a side note, this Overt Fence stance is almost exactly the same position recommended for walking or standing when in dangerously overcrowded situations, where there is a crowd stampede for example in a sports show or music concert. There was a mass stampede during Halloween on the streets of Seoul in South Korea in 2022. Over 150 people were crushed to death during the ruckus - mostly because they had fallen to the ground and were trampled on. There was no real reason why it happened. Shoppers just started running, some fell, and the mass just continued running over them. The Fence is the best position to be in to stop you hitting the deck when you don't want to. It is also recommended as the position if you're in an earthquake and has been tested and proven to withstand forces from all angles. It is the best position to keep you on your feet. That's not just me and Geoff T saying it, but science itself.

The Fence is that good!

RIGHT HAND, CLYDE

I have watched hundreds, if not thousands, of videos of CCTV footage of assaults (and I don't ever want to see another one until the day I return back to the ether, but I'm digressing). What I saw is that pretty much any time a man hits anyone it is going to be with his right hand and it is likely to be a hooking shot. This is often the first shot. **The right hand hook**. He will follow up from there but if you can anticipate that first shot, prevent it or move out of the way, then you are already on your way to lowering his abilities to strike you.

SAY "NO" TWICE.
THREE IS TOO MANY ALREADY

If you are in conversation at this early Stage you need to watch how many times you have said 'NO'.

If you have said or indicated the word 'NO' twice in any way at all - 'No, I don't need your help right now, thank you.', 'No, I won't give you my phone number because I don't know you. Sorry,' or any other way where you have refused twice and are now being pressured to say it the third time then you've got a situation on your hands.

Although this particular man may not have bad intent, the fact is that those who commit the really bad crimes of sexual assault always bypass your 'NO' more than twice.

If you've had to say 'NO' twice and he's not taken the hint, then you should really take note, become stronger within yourself and more resistant. Depending on where you are, there is a likelihood the situation is going to turn physical.

You should also be ready for this person to follow you wherever you are going, so now is the time to make sure you don't walk him into your home or into the communal area of the flats you live in. It is time to wake up even more to the fact this person is real threat and a supreme manipulator, a trickster, and you don't want to be alone with him.

It might be that he is not that, and is just an annoying man, but he is also showing the same signs as the really Bad Guys so I think it is better to take the safer option.

Again, it's not about being paranoid. It's about having the right knowledge so you can take action early and not get caught out. Just knowing this makes you more alert to the situation and that's always a good thing.

Note that adrenaline will probably kick in and start affecting your body in powerful ways as soon as you realise you're under threat. So use that to your advantage should things kick off.

Have a think now about what actions you would take in such a situation where you've said "NO" twice and he's still pushing you.

AVOID, DISSUADE,
THEN HIT THE CRAZY SWITCH

The best advice is, where possible, to avoid him and avoid all conflict. Get away if you can. Don't engage if that's possible, or at least break engagement quickly.

That's true for physical engagement as well as verbal.

Use short sentences with nothing he can use to continue the conversation.

Next, or at the same time, you need to deter him. You do that by moving to a busier location. You do that by putting up your Covert Fences and preventing him from getting to you physically.

And if that doesn't work, and you're in danger, then you need to switch on the crazy.

You've given him every chance to leave you alone, but he's not and your limbs or life are on the line. How much do you want to keep your life or limbs? If you really want to keep them you're going to have to switch on the crazy.

We can all be enlightened beings and display our veneer of civilised social etiquette. But I've seen it fade many times when the poop smashed the fan. When it comes to survival the animal comes out. It never went anywhere anyway. You were just holding it back because the world required us to. Give it a strong enough pinch and out comes that animal.

I remember a tiny little virus not long ago. People bought excessive loads of toilet paper for no obvious reason. Maybe they were going to eat it? They even fought each over that toilet paper in supermarkets. Civility gone, because of a few rolls of toilet paper.

So you might need to drop your civility when your life in on the line. You gave the Bad Guy the opportunity to go away. You tried to dissuade him, you tried to avoid him, but he was insistent. He's left you no choice. He's made the decision for you. He's going to hurt you too. So, you gotta do what you gotta do.
So hit the crazy switch and save your life.

HIT HIM BEFORE HE HITS YOU?

Can you hit first?

This is a moral as well as legal question.

The answer is that if you feel like you need to **immediately** protect yourself and any valuable property then you should hit first and hit really hard. Hit as many shots as it takes to get the job done. In other words don't stop until the threat is neutralised and/or you can walk away safely.

You do not need to stay around to admire your shot and assess its effectiveness and you do not need to stay around to fight more.

Hit.
And run.

Stun and run too. If you hit them and they're stunned then you can often run.

The legal term for hitting first is the 'Pre-Emptive Strike'. With regards the legal side for your country please seek advice. This is just guidance being provided here and it does not take your legal responsibilities into account.

However, your moral right to hit someone first who is going to harm you, does not change. It's stood the test of time, been around for ever. If someone is going to hit you, then you have societal agreement that you can hit them first. We've all agreed that. Ask anyone you know.

The moral right to do so is a duty to protect yourself and no one can say it is wrong.

Note that I highlighted the word 'immediately' at the top. To hit someone you must be under threat right now. If the person is walking away from the situation and will no longer be a threat but you chase them down to give them a good hiding, that is not a pre-emptive strike. You can hit them if you are genuinely under threat, not because you're a martial artist or ninja or you feel as if they deserve it. However, if the person walking away is still a threat then you can hit them. Maybe they are walking away to get a weapon. Maybe they are leaving to hurt someone else you love in the next room. That makes them still at threat to you or a loved one and you are still justified to hit them.

So if you're genuinely under threat, and you feel that you have to hit to stop that threat, then you should hit to stop that threat. It is a moral duty to protect yourself (or protect someone else who is in imminent danger).

If you are justified in hitting him, because you were in fear, it will be the extent of how much you hurt the Bad Guy that can be up for debate later, maybe in court.

But hey, apologies for being facetious, but you can only answer questions in court if you're alive, right?

So if someone just says hello to you and you know they had no intention of harming you then you can't just kill them or smack them because they were annoying you. That's not allowed. That's not self defence and that will be difficult to explain to a jury and judge.

But if you have a genuinely held belief that you will be harmed, and you are in a situation which is genuinely dangerous to you, or will become dangerous if you don't act right now, then you have the right to stop that person from harming you.

Stopping them can include killing them on this occasion if that is the most suitable way to stop them right now from harming you.

But do check the laws of your location.

Just for reference, I've found judges to be quite intelligent and understanding people. I'm happy to go to court and explain my actions to them, so don't be fearful of them. Just make sure they know why you did what you did. Court is not like in the movies. You can usually talk to the judge if you ask politely.

But you can only go to court if you're still alive so the pre-emptive strike is a major tool you need to get in your toolbox.

STAGE THREE
THE EARLY FIGHT

Now the fight is on. It has just started.

He's gone to grab you or he's actually got hold of you.

Or he's hit you - and things will now continue progressing from here or you might get a break if you trained for it or get lucky.

You're in a land of confusion now. A mish-mash of things can happen.

But even in this land of confusion there are only a set number of things he can do.

He has only the body of a human and that's all he can use to get at you. Understanding what he can do allows us to come out of a world of total confusion into a more orderly place where we can can fight him off. Knowing what can happen allows us to intercept his moves as soon as he starts them. To him it will feel like whatever he tries is failing. He won't be used to that, won't be used to his 'victim' being one step ahead, ready to deal with him.

To be one step ahead though takes knowledge and training. So we are going to build that knowledge and blend it with the best skills of all time - but you will have to do the training! I can't do it for you, unfortunately. Just knowing what is in this book takes you a huge way towards defending yourself. But training and practice - actually doing the skills - puts the icing on this sweet pie that we are going to hit Bad Guy with in his face.

What is often most confusing at this Stage is that there appear to be endless possibilities that can be used against us and that we could use. To some level, that is true but the fact is that the basics, the fundamentals of any technique or position, are all the same and so when we know these we can start simplifying everything.

Let's talk about grabs as an example. How many ways can someone grab you? Have a quick think about it right now. It's an absolute tonne, isn't it! But isn't a grab just a grab? Isn't it just him using his hand to grab something of yours? Yes, it is! To grab he has to close his fingers and squeeze. Doesn't really matter much if it's our clothes or our limbs that he's grabbed (hair is different though and we'll deal with that later). And so it is with grabs that we only need to understand a couple of principles of escaping them and we can pretty much escape all of them.

This is one place where I differ in my approach from most martial arts and self defence coaches. They tend to teach a hundred techniques but rarely the actual main principle. I think it is because they just don't know or they just don't seek the principles, the underlying concepts. I think I learned the hard way because I really had to. I couldn't afford to flick through my mental library of ten thousand grab escapes when someone grabbed me. My job was intense and to survive I didn't have that luxury whilst someone tried to drag me into a road and under a bus on Harrow Road, which actually happened to someone else. Trying to figure out how to do this or how to do that was going to get me hurt in live situations against some of the most savvy violent men in London. Guys who had practised this lifestyle since birth and knew what they were doing. And so I veered towards thinking in principles and concepts. Actually I didn't do it on purpose. My brain just figured it out and I had plenty of eureka moments, which have led to what is in this book. I wish coaches had told me these principles when I first started martial arts because they would have saved me thousands of hours of training! I could have learned to play the piano AND climbed Kilimanjaro by now!

But in the martial arts the instructors tend not to have that real need for survival. They're training in safe environments, in the dojo or wrestling mats, and losing is not going to get them killed. Very few of them have to actually use the skills in reality and even fewer will do it at the frequency or quantity that I did. I worked years in teams that dealt with excessively violent and anti-social people. It was a speciality of mine and I was chosen as the assistant others picked to go along with them if they thought the situation might get a bit tasty. So I went along, at first because it allowed me to continuously test my skills against live and ungiving individuals and then later I went along because I knew I could do the job better than others and so I was the best help to my colleagues who needed it. I became the go-to guy, the port of call to go along if they needed a job done quickly but preferably without violence. I never went because I wanted to be more involved in violence and anger and aggression. I sought other routes and always tried to find the non- physical solutions but there are those people who only want to do one thing and that's to use their physicality, and I happened to have a good understanding of how to restrict them with that so less people were harmed overall. In fourteen years in police service, I arrested hundreds of people and assisted in the physical detention in hundreds of others, and I never had a single notice against me for harming anyone beyond the standard bruises you'd get in any scramble you take part in.

So we are going to work here on principles that can be applied at a wider level so you have less to remember but more ability at the same time. You're going to be freed up to think your own things too. Learning principles allows you to think on your feet and you can invent your own ways to do things when the need arises. Just as importantly though, you're going to reduce confusion and get skills that are going to help you escape early, before things get really deep.

Hey, because this is called the Early Fight does not make it any less dangerous than the Deep Fight (in Stage Four). You can get hurt here just as much as you can in Stage Four. The main difference between these two stages is tactical. To escape in the Deep Fight will take longer and require a lot more technical knowledge of techniques, some of which have several moves in them to make them work. So the skills start to become a little more complicated to do in Stage Four.

At this stage, Stage Three: The Early Fight, you might be lucky and break away after one good hit or one good shove. At this stage we are still on our feet and he hasn't fully got control of us like he would if we were on the floor, with him on top.

We are most likely going back and forth in our struggle, where for moments he is in control of the situation and in some moments we get control back. But we haven't lost control more substantially. After this we enter Stage Four (the Deep Fight) where he maybe has taken us to the floor or he's got a full strangle on us and is choking us etcetera. It's a very scary thing the Deep Fight - IF you don't know what happens there.

A good thing about the Deep Fight is that very few attackers know how to fight there. In all the things I've seen on the street and of all the times I've dealt with people on the ground, I've never met anyone who knows how to fight on the floor. Big Guys become upturned turtles on the ground. Everyone can hit and punch. And everyone can use force to hold you down. But the minute you start to know how to deal with someone on the floor you bypass all those things.

But that's all a little later. Right now, here in the Early Fight, and things are still very dangerous. You can be dragged somewhere, you can be hit and hurt or knocked out, or you can rapidly be taken into the Deep.

We want to deter him and stop him right here. So let's work on that first.

DON'T GET DRAGGED

You really don't want to be on the ground, no matter how much jiu jitsu you've done. Doesn't matter if your instructor thinks it's the best martial art in the world and tells you it is the fastest growing.

I'm not slating jiu jitsu because I really do love the art form as well as the competition of it, but it is currently marketed as self defence, not just self defence but as the "best one ever of all time eternity". And I like to remind those who say such silly things that Rickson Gracie - considered by many in the know, including Chuck Norris, Joe Rogan and the entire infamous Gracie clan themselves - says jiu jitsu is about 20% self defence and becoming even less as it becomes more competition focused over time.

So I am going to repeat what I've said for a very long time - do not purposely take a situation to the ground unless you really really have to. You want to avoid the ground as much as you can.

Do not listen to what jiu jitsu instructors and online tutorials are saying again and again to do. In fact do the opposite and stay standing, and I'll show you how.

This is the case if it's a man against a man but even more so for a woman against a man. Don't go to the ground!

But that doesn't mean you won't find yourself there. So you do have to prepare for it, preferably even excel at it.

So how can Bad Guy get you to the floor when you didn't want to go there?

It could be that you were dragged to the floor.

It could be that you slipped or tripped and ended up there. Or it could be that you were thrown.

That's it.

The statistically most likely time you're going to find yourself on the floor is when someone is trying to rob you and you fight them. It could be a bag snatcher or phone snatcher and he's after your property but you fought back. Next thing, you slip or he fights back and you lose your balance and you're on the floor. He might even purposely push you and you find yourself on the floor like an upturned turtle with your eyes rolling around inside your head. I'm not saying that to be funny but it actually will be just like that. When you first hit the floor, if you haven't spent time training there, it is a disorientating place. It's important to know this. That's why you're going to have to spend a little time there and get familiar with it.

A robber has no vested interest in you personally, only your property, so he'll just leave when you're on the floor. Taking his chance to get away. He might hit you one for good measure but that's about it.

In a property-snatch situation, in a snatch-and-run in other words, again only a malicious attacker will throw you. The only reason he is likely to fight is to get your property. And so the only reason you end up on the floor is because you tried to prevent him from taking it and clung to it, and so he used more force and you ended up on the floor.

I am not saying you should not fight back, but just pointing out the facts here.

(Personally, as sad as it is to let them win, I would say you want to let them take the property and avoid the physical levels of the altercation. You might get hurt physically as well as emotionally. Better to call the police asap. You may never get your property back but you won't have to deal with the long psychological effects of having had a fight, and you won't have any of the injuries that come with physical confrontations. Sorry to tell you this but it's my best advice on the subject having dealt with it on a personal and professional level too.

So the robber has no real vested interest in you individually, and so the interaction is likely to be very brief.

The more serious offences such as sexual assaults and domestic violence, tend to be more prolonged than robberies. In those cases you are more likely to be grabbed and shoved about for various reasons. The man is trying to dominate you, trying to get you to obey. He could be using force to try to move you to another location where he is safer. In those kinds of scenarios you are more likely to either trip accidentally and fall to the ground or you will be purposely pushed or dragged to the ground by the Bad Guy.

So the first most important thing to stop you from hitting the ground is structure and balance.

To have good balance means you must have the correct base to start with.

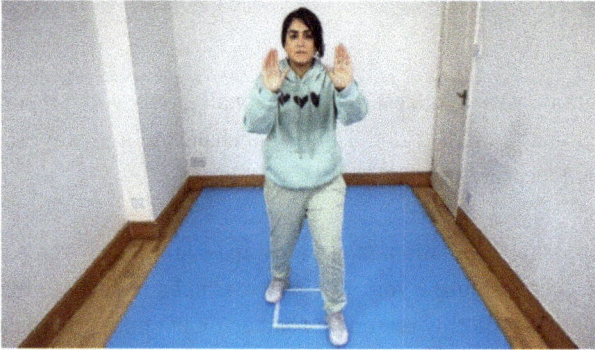

The Fence gives you this base. I would really like it if you actually got into the Fence yourself now, or soon, and copied this so you understand it better. Please acknowledge at least four Brownie points from me if you're doing it right now.

Here you see Rahilla is standing with her feet on a square. This is basically how your feet should be. They should be a comfortable distance, about shoulder width apart. Same distance forwards as they are wide from one another. Making a square shape. This is the shape that gives you stability in every direction. You are more stable as you stand and more stable as you move about. It allows you to resist and fight off being pushed or pulled from any direction.

So get this position.

Remember your hands are at about neck height, about shoulder width apart. Arms are not straight but also not fully bent; ready to push but also ready to accept forces pushing them back. Springy in other words.

Both feet point forwards (ish) but at a comfortable position. They don't have to be dead straight. Be relaxed. Hips are pretty much square on, which is the position that allows you to generate most force forwards and to resist anyone pushing you or pulling you away.

(A sideways stance, like in standard martial arts and boxing, is not well designed for preventing push and pull forces)..

Remember The Fence is a 'ready' position - you need to be ready to move or hit or fight from it.

So check in your head. Are ready to and able to move? Nice and springy. Are you ready to push? Ready to resist being pulled, ready to block, ready to move out of the way? To hit first or move out of the way and hit back?

Consider that a checklist. You need to go over it. Please do it many times. Let it become part of you over time.

We will add movement and we'll practice in a while, but for now I don't want to digress. Let's build one major skill at a time.

Just remember that you will be pressing down with the midfoot or balls of your feet rather than your heels, as that allows you to remain springy and ready to move.

Now, if you've had a go at that, let's move on.

When you are pushed or pulled or dragged, you really need to widen your stance.

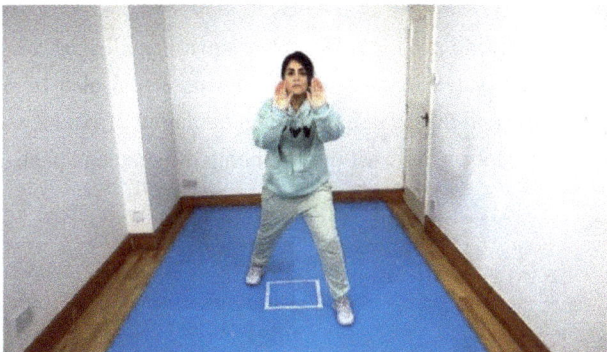

Notice how Rahilla's feet are now outside the square, but still equal length apart in all directions to keep that stable square shape. She has also bent her legs. And dropped her hips down a little more.

If you are being pushed or pulled too strongly, you can go more flat footed, to get a better grip on the floor with your feet. (But to be mobile you will need to be pressing down with the balls or midfoot more).

You are now in what we will call the Wide Fence.

Note how in the next photo Bad Guy is trying to drag Rahilla away and she has dropped her hips even lower. Whilst maintaining a strong structure, she is able to fight back and resist better.

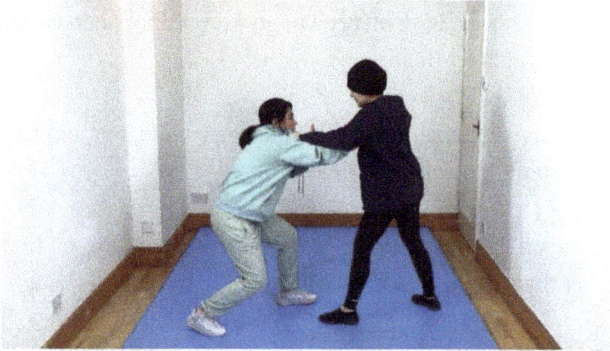

You would probably do something like this automatically anyway but I wanted to make sure you were aware of it so you can deploy it when you choose rather than only doing it on automatic. This will I help you sharpen your instincts even more.

If Rahilla had stayed upright and kept her square small she would have been far easier to drag away (as in pics below). There would also be an increased likelihood of tripping and falling due to her feet being out of balance, so she could easily end up on the floor just by tripping or being dragged and pushed.

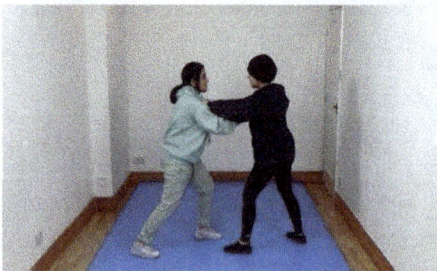

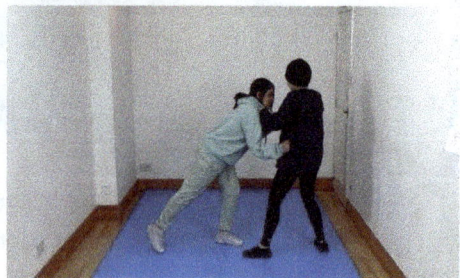

The same applies if someone grabs you from the rear. If you stay upright and with a narrow stance you will be much easier to pull away and you can lose your balance and end up on the floor.

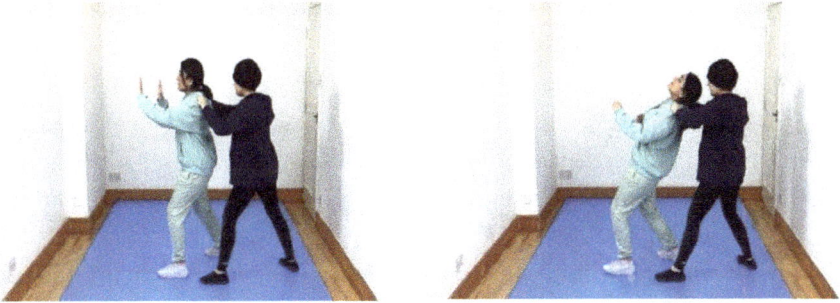

But if you can widen your stance and drop your hips lower than his then you have the chance of being in a better position to resist and start the fight back.

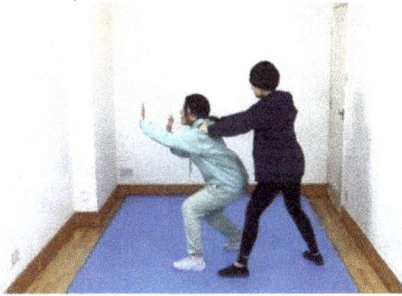

Of course you are not going to stay in these positions like you've turned into a statue. You might be in them for a second, get pulled, lose your footing, gain your footing back, accidentally go upright, then gain balance and drop your hips and resist again.

In a fight situation there is going to be a lot of movement, some of it is to your advantage and some of it is not.

However, in practice, you need to make sure you train gently for a while. Learn the moves. Do not apply pressure to them if it's not going to develop you. Make sure your training partner knows they are there to help you, not to push you to fail but to allow you to learn at the correct pace.

Practice.

Get into The Fence. (Choose the Overt or Covert. You should practice both anyway)

Your partner stands in front and they pull you (at the shoulder or clothing)
You resist them by dropping your hips and widening your stance. (Getting into the Wide Fence in other words).

What you might find is that they surprise you and initially move you a step or two but as soon as you manage to get that Wide Fence shape, you now start to be quite difficult to move about. From here you can fight or break away if you can.

Now get them to push you and do all the same again. (Last time they pulled you, remember?)
Next they go behind and do all the above again. Start with pulls, and resist them. Then move to pushes and resist them. Get your balance and get control.

You are now starting to become drag and push proof! Yippee!

To practice on your own.
Start in the normal Fence position.
Imagine someone in front has grabbed you and is going to drag you away.
Adjust your stance, drop your hips and use them to pull back so you can't be pulled away. Make sure your structure is strong. Practice doing this (from 1-3) several times.
Next imagine they are going to push you and repeat the same practice as above.
Now imagine someone is behind you and do the same practice (1-4 above) as if someone is pulling or pushing you from behind.

These practices are better with a partner because they can take you off balance and unravel your Fence shape, so you have to keep fighting to get it back. But there are benefits of practising on your own too. You get to learn the shape better and you can focus on you thought pattern and emotions. If you're practising on your own you need to get inside your head a little more, but also feel what your body is doing. Have a few practices and then let's move on to working how to not get thrown next!

DON'T GET THROWN

As has been said before, The Fence is the best position to remain standing and to fight from. Beyond that you need to have good footwork so that if you are dragged or pushed you can regain your balance quickly.

Another thing you need to know is how to get off the floor quickly should you fall. To do that you need to know the amazingly titled technique called The Stand Up.

We are going to practice these things in a short while, build up to them, but right now it is essential for you to know that you could also end up on the floor if you are 'thrown' there.

Some throws come naturally to us as humans. You can even see schoolboys doing these in the playground without ever having any training.

The most common and natural to us is the leg trip and the second most common is some form of a headlock throw. Here you can see Rahilla using the leg trip to throw the Bad Guy down.

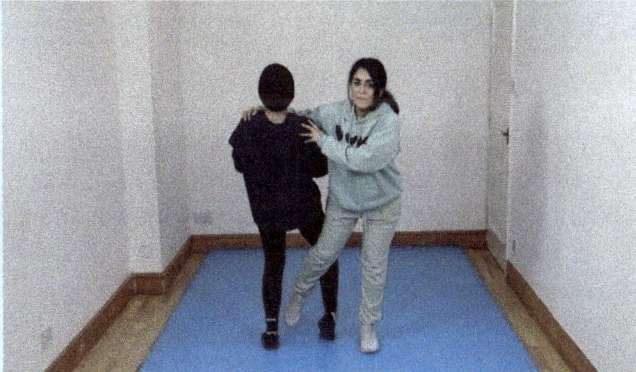

The leg trip throw is one which all schoolboys use naturally. You may have seen this or variations of it. The official judo name is *osoto gari*, roughly meaning 'large reaping of the leg'.

The second most likely 'throw' is the headlock throw. You can see Rahilla using it here to take down the Bad Guy.

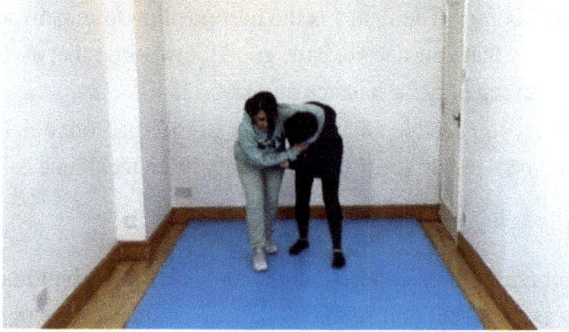

And it tends to continue until you are on the floor in a headlock position.

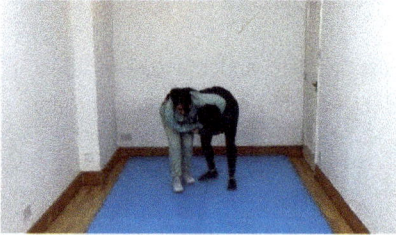

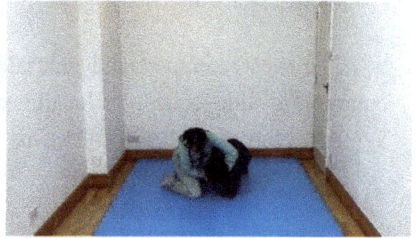

If you want to see them in action, just type 'Osoto Gari judo' or 'Major Outer Reap judo' into a search engine for the leg trip and 'Koshi Guruma judo' or 'headlock throw' for videos of the headlock throw. You will find many variations of them there. Just be aware that in reality they won't be quite so tidy as they look in demonstrations.

These are throws that you might even revert to yourself and so have a practice at them if you can get a couple of judo mats.

Beyond these two he is just likely to drag/push you somewhere or use some bastardised version of a throw he's put together on the spot. It's very unlikely he knows how to do proper throws from judo or wrestling. I have a half-decent background in both and I have to say that in all the physical altercations I have been involved in not a single one knew how to throw me. Not one. I was genuinely surprised by that. After all, in judo classes almost everyone could throw me and so for three times a week, for a long time, I'd encountered people who'd have a good go at it. Funny how in judo and wrestling classes so many people could throw me, isn't it?!

The other side of the coin is that having taken at least a hundred criminals to the floor myself (and getting a reputation for doing so amongst my colleagues), I can genuinely say only four people didn't go down first

attempt. Every single other person went to the floor immediately.

(I'll just tell you that of those who didn't go down easily one was a professional athlete in her prime fitness, another was a paranoid schizophrenic in full disorder mode, and two others were just very strong gym- bunnies, who were on cocaine. The reason I didn't manage to throw them was through my own choice. They were fighting so hard that they were going to hurt themselves if they landed with their heads on the concrete floor with me on top. It was easier to continue fighting them until they were tired and then I could gently take them down, which I did on each occasion).

So, very few people know how to throw and very few know how to stop being thrown.

For your information, if you can make time and really want to become unthrowable then go and do judo or wrestling twice a week for a couple of months. Your aim won't be to learn how to throw your opponent in loads of different ways - that can take a while - your aim is to learn how NOT to get thrown but also how it feels to get thrown when it happens. It can be quite winding. The first time when the air is knocked out of your lungs, you'll know what I mean!

In judo (and wrestling) you will learn and practice what is called 'breakfalls'. These are skills that teach you how to soften the blow of a fall and so are really useful to learn. They can't be coached in a book but you can search them online or attend a class and learn.

In the meantime, here are the two biggest secrets to not getting thrown: knowledge and attitude.

Knowledge: Knowing that he might try to throw you, knowing that you might get tripped, is empowering and allows you to potentially stop it before it happens. It also prepares you in case you do get thrown, making it less shocking in reality. You might just jump right back to your feet when it happens too, because you were expecting it as a possibility.

Attitude. Thinking and saying to yourself, "No, you're not going to throw me, buddy," adds *massive* resilience to your ability to resist being thrown. It really does. So if someone grabs you, you need to think something like that (or "No, you're not going to drag me away", or, "No, you're not going to move me easily, pal.")

You will become stronger in yourself. Sounds silly but it really works. It's how professional fighters think. A third of all fighting is the mental game. You only win if you think you're going to win. You're less likely to win if you think you won't.

Anyway, you're going to continue learning how to not hit the deck and you're going to have those skills under your belt as you continue through this book.

Just one thing before we move on, when someone does try to throw you, no matter how they try to throw you, dropping your hips below theirs, and creating a strong structure with your body to push against them, will often render a throw useless. It really will.

It's the same position as not being dragged/pushed away. You already know it and I will be sending you a short video via email about it to make sure you know how to do it properly.

HE'S HITTING YOU. WHAT IS HAPPENING?

When a man hits a woman he usually grabs her first and then hits her, or he hits and then grabs and continues hitting from there. There is usually a grab involved with being hit when it comes to a women being attacked. This is a control mechanism again.

It is rarely like that when two men start to fight. They face each other and let punches fly. They only grab when they are overwhelmed by the other man's punches. Men fight that way for many reasons, including ego and competitiveness, which are not relevant for us here in this book because when a woman is attacked by a man it is a power issue and he wants to dominate and take control. So it will be really rare for a man take a woman on and stand facing her like in marital arts and fighting competitions.

Note how men will square up and so it is a challenge that both men choose to take part in, even if one is the aggressor and the other is not. With a woman the man will not square up, face off or challenge her to a 'fair' chivalrous fight like he's living in medieval ages.

Men also like to fight when there's an audience. When their mates can see how macho they are.

When a woman is attacked, the man doesn't really want anyone seeing him beating a woman. That won't do his ego any good. And anyway, the intentions when hitting a woman are different to when hitting a man.

So he will likely grab at some stage. But he is equally as likely to hit first and then grab.

So you have The Fence already up. You should be in it, with your arms up ready to fight off any grabs and ready to block off any punches.

However, you also need to stay out of his reach. That is the best thing to do. Move away, far enough that he can't get to you. That is the best place to be. Fence or not: Be far away. If he can lean forward and grab you then he's too close already.

Let's get to the nitty-gritty. With regards being hit, the best defence is offence.

You need to be hitting him, kicking him, scratching him, biting him and doing everything you can to fight him off. This is indirect fighting of course. To directly try to stop him hitting you is not that easy. With a tonne of practice you can do it to a reasonable level - you might be able to deflect his punch or parry it or block it like they do in martial arts and the movies, but the reality is that it's seriously not that easy to do. It takes years and years of practice and often requires some decent level of athleticism to avoid being hit or to block it off, especially when he's a tonne bigger than you and has grabbed you and is trying to drag you about like a rag doll.

If you watch sports fighting competitions you'll see that the one thing they do when an onslaught comes their way is to move away from it. If they can't, then they cover up until they find a moment to hit back and then they move out of the way.

You are starting to get into the realms of the Deep Fight now if he's grabbing and hitting you, and you will need to bring all your skills and knowledge into play. Use every trick in the book. Hit him everywhere. Bite anything. Scratch anything.

So keep moving and keep doing anything you can if he grabs you or hits you. We will come back to this to cover how to escape grabs of various kinds, but right now, you can fight back using what we've said here.

One extra point you should know about being hit is that, obviously, it can be very painful but unless it is totally debilitating, you can ride through it. It's just pain. It's not nice but if it isn't enough damage to stop you then you will have to work through it.

I've been hit a lot and my first thought, like it is for most fighters, is "Is that pain or injury?"

If it's just pain we accept it and carry on (and I might use that to anger myself too). If it's an injury we try to rapidly figure out what it is so we can work around it to carry on. If it's debilitating and I am in too much pain to function, well, then I just do what I have to do in the situation. I might curl up to get my breath back for example, but I know I will be coming back. In a self defence situation, I will do what I have to do. To live.

Women are much better at dealing with pain than men anyway. Some of you get it every month and some go through child birth. The only real reason you might struggle with pain in a self defence situation is psychological, because you are not used to the situation that the pain is coming from and you don't know when this will be over or even if it will be over. In reality, if it's just pain, most of you can handle it better than I probably could.

But if he's hitting you, fight back and move out of the way regardless of pain or injuries. You don't have any choice. It's what you'll have to do.

CAN *YOU* HIT HIM?

I don't mean do you need permission to hit him. I mean can you actually do the act of hitting him.

Are you able to hit him, in reality, and effect him?

You probably have your own ideas with regards this. You're probably going to punch him. Women in our surveys, and my friends, seem to incline towards an elbow or a punch. The other one is a knee (or kick) to the groin. That's all good. We're going to enhance all that for you and make these moves truly powerful. You're going to use them anyway so let's make them multitudes better, shall we.

But   first…

Let's be real.

An attacker is expecting every single one of the above things to happen.

He knows you're going to go for his groin or going to elbow him or punch him. He's going to be ready for it. He has prepared for you to fight back. So you really do need to up your game with this.

I'm not going to help you. There's nothing I can do for you here.

Just kidding!!

You're really going to make a dent in him when you hit him. But just before we learn about *how* to hit we need to know *where* to hit him for maximum effect.

Let's look at where he is most vulnerable.

WHERE TO HURT HIM: THE TARGETS!

Before we cover how to hit maximally we're going to figure out where to hit. I know, I know, you just want to hit things and that's far more interesting than learning boring things like where to hit. And I know this is not the usual way this is done. Very few actually teach targets. Very few. They teach how to hit and then leave you to it.

But once you know where to hit, it frees you up massively. You become far more effective.

For example, you know you can hit to the groin. Most of you would just go for it with a knee or kick. But you can hit the area with other things too You can elbow it. You can punch it. You can stamp on it. You can headbutt it. This is worth knowing.

That one target can be hit in so many ways!

Headbutt, did I say?
Yes.
Remember you could be on the floor. You can and should still hit people when you're on the floor.

In fact if you're kneeling you can pretty much do all the same things that you can do when you're standing.

So maybe you're kneeling, and he's either standing, kneeling or on the floor. You can do to him from your kneeling position pretty much most of what you can do when you're standing, and you have pretty much the same targets available to go for too. I bet you didn't know that – that what you can do standing you can pretty much do if you find yourself kneeling.

When standing you might have kicked him in the groin. Now you're kneeling but he is standing - you could headbutt or punch his groin. If he's on the ground you could still hit him there.

If the groin presents itself. You must deliver to it more accurately than a UPS parcel flung at your letterbox.

So by knowing targets we free up the ability to hit him more creatively.

Another thing you need to understand are the genuine effects of hitting specific targets.

To hurt him you most likely need to deliver a lot of force to an area. One way of doing that is to hit the same area as many times as you can, so you get accumulated impact.

In reality you need to keep hitting wherever you can until you know you are safe. But if you can hit one target many times then that's an added Brucie Bonus and will really break him down.

Otherwise just hit as hard as you can and as often as you can, wherever you can.

The ideal way to hit is to hit whatever he has presented to you. Hit it as hard as you can and then as many times as you can. That's what you need to do.

When a target presents itself to you, say, 'Thank you,' and crack it.

It is quite difficult to choose your target or set it up if you're not versed and practised in such a thing. So hit what he gives you to hit.

A little later we'll cover how to send someone unconscious and other dangerous attacks. Just remember that you don't have to kill someone in every situation. There are gradations of what you need to do or what you are willing to do in any given situation but the final decision is yours. Only you are there at the time and only you know what level of force your brain is telling you to use right now. You are on your own to make those decisions at the time. Your brain is a clever thing though so I would take note of what it's saying and make decisions around that.

When you hit someone these are some of the effects you can have:

You create pain:
To which he shows no reaction;
To which he gets angry and fights even harder; To which he reacts and backs off.

You incapacitate him:
For a very short period of time, in which case he will resume where he left off once he recovers; You incapacitate him fully, making him unable to continue at all.

You do not stop him but you distract him from what he was doing, giving you a chance to escape his technique, or get away or hit him. For example he is strangling you so you punch him in the eye. It might not have connected properly but it's enough to distract him, giving you a chance to escape and shout for help.

So here are some targets you can aim for. You know where each of these is so I don't really need to include a picture with arrows pointing at bodyparts! But as you go through please take an extra moment to remember where each of these is so it becomes embedded into your mind.

THE FEET

They're worth a good foot stomp at the top of his foot or on his toes, especially if you've got strong heels on your footwear. Realistically this move will just irritate the attacker but it gives him something to think about and shows you are fighting back. The best use of the foot stomp is not as a move by itself though. Use it to do other things. Use it to distract him from what you're really about to do. As he's moving his foot, and his mind is focused on that, you could hit him, bite him, poke him or do what you need for your given situation. It might be that he releases his grip enough that you can fight out of it . It could be that the foot stomp causes him to open his legs wider so now you can attack his groin. The foot stomp is a distraction rather than a fight finisher.

THE SHIN

If you've got some solid shoes the shin is worth a kick. It will hurt. Scraping a shoe sole down the shin is also going to hurt. Again, it is a distraction technique mostly, just like the foot stomp is.

THE THIGH

From a standing point of view, as an untrained non-martial artist, there is nothing really effective you can do to the thigh. However, when close up, or on the ground, and his clothing allows it, you can reach the inner thigh, grab and squeeze or pinch the skin and flesh as hard as you can, and you're likely to get a reaction. You could even bite this area if you're in place to do so. You can scratch deep. The thigh, especially the inner thigh, has a lot of nerves and they are likely to react to an attack in that area if you can get to the skin. Of course a key or pen digging into that area would also make that leg move and you can potentially try something else while he reacts.

THE GROIN

Kicking or kneeing a man in the groin/testicles/penis is nothing like you think it is. Sorry. It is not like in the movies or how you imagine it to be. I need you to know this so you are better prepared and more able to use that target to full effect.

I've been training in the martial arts long enough to see many many men get hit in the groin, often by accident and sometimes by less than accident.

I've been hit in the groin more times than I'd like and I've hit guys in the groin too. On two occasions they were debilitated and on one occasion the guy went unconscious when I hit him. But not in the manner you currently think he did. Not like in the movies. He actually walked around for a minute or two and only after that did he collapse to the floor and pass out. It wasn't even a hard shot either. I'd just been 'lucky' to hit all the right dangling bits. I felt so bad about it because he was actually a really nice guy and my shot was careless and accidental.

So the first thing to note is that when a man is hit in the groin properly, with a solid connection to the right parts there might be a paused moment where he can't/won't do anything. A sort of temporary paralysis. It is often a phase when he's contemplating what has just happened, assessing what the consequences will be that will flood up his body any second now. He's usually not in pain during this time though. It is after this pause that he could be in so much pain that he is incapable of doing anything. The pain isn't sudden. It is a rising pain. It's first not there, and the man is waiting, seeing if it is coming. Then it appears and it rises sharply in severity.

But I have also seen men who can override being hit in the groin, and I guess that was because the shot missed the target or was just not powerful enough. And on these occasions they come back very angry. I have seen this happen, where the man was hit in the groin, stopped for literally a second, assessed and decided that he was okay, then came back doubly angry and extremely violently…but after a few punches at the 'victim' the man stopped again due to the pain. Had he connected during that time, the 'victim' would have been in real trouble.

The point that I am making is that a good groin strike will stop a man, but be ready for him to come back at you for a bit too. If he has collapsed then that is perfect, but if he is still standing then be wary.

Either way, that reaction, to assess the situation, and the short pause whilst he moves his hands to his groin, which is often his immediate response, can give you enough time to hit him again or get away.

If you're going for the groin area, here's something you really should do - hit him so hard that you hit right through the groin area. If you are going to kick or knee his groin, you need to understand that you need to drive right through the area, as if you want your knee to pass all the way through right up to his bellybutton. That's what you should be doing for several reasons. Firstly – though less importantly right now - because that's the way you are supposed to do all strikes. All hitting action requires you to hit right through the target as much as you can and not just hit on the surface. Flicking the testicles might hurt him or it might just tickle him. But sending your knee up there so they are as flat as a pancake, and travelling up to his bellybutton, well, that's a different story you'll be telling your mates when you get home for tea and macaron.But the most important reason you hit through the groin area is that you can then also connect to all those other nerves and things that are hanging about near the testicles. The whole area there is quite susceptible to pains. So I say that when you kick with your shin, drive it up really really high into his body so you collect his entire nether regions and navel area and make it move up to his bellybutton. All those extra nerves will now also be tingling, not just the few in the genitals. That's how you should be hitting that area. That way he is less likely to come at you after the short pause and he will go to sleepy-byes. You can keep hitting him if the situation requires or you can walk away. Below is how to do a groin snap-kick, which is the move you'd probably consider doing anyway. I just want to make sure you've got it so it makes him squeal sharper than a piggy.

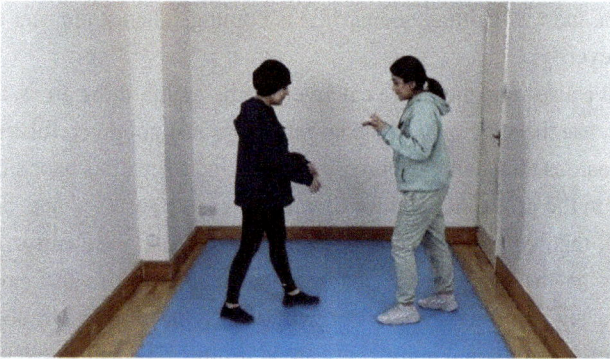

As you do the groin kick, first lift your knee up powerfully in the direction of the Bad Guy's groin.

Keep that knee lifting!

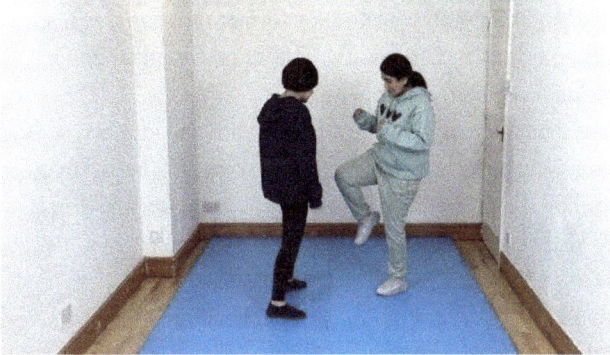

Then you snap that shin and lower part of the leg.

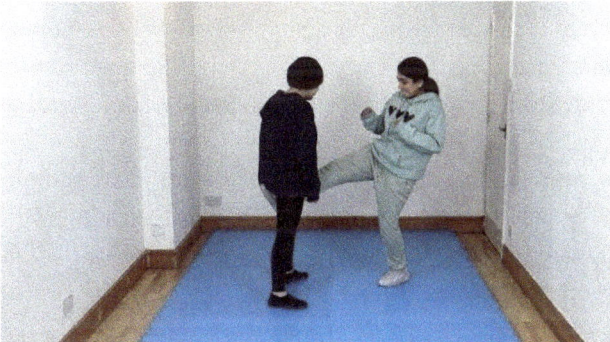

So that it whips right up, as shown here.

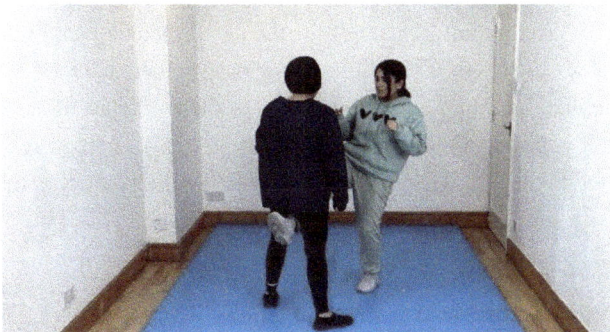

Note how it's the shin that has connected rather than the foot. This is the correct way to do it. This means your shin bone will connect and gather up all the goodies and send them towards the heavens, rather than your foot, which is much softer. It also means that should he move backwards or forwards, you still have a chance of catching him with your foot or further up your shin respectively. If you just aim with your foot and he moves, you're pretty much going to lose the shot. So focus on delivering that shin to him.

Reminder that you really do need to kick hard and kick upwards as if you want your foot to end up, or even travel beyond towards his head. If you manage to get your foot coming out of the top of his head, that should stop him for a minute and ask to speak to his mamma.

Nice.

He deserves it. We're not going to do this kind of thing for fun. We're only going to do it for things we think are serious. But if his intent is on harming us, then we have the right to defend ourselves, and I say a moral duty to do so too.

In light of that, don't forget that in some situations the groin area will not be accessible for kicks but might be for other actions. You can bite the area or grab and yank bits of it or even repeatedly stab it with a key or pen or brush end. The choice is yours and depends on where you are at the time: standing or on the ground, and depends how severe the situation is and what you feel you should do to survive.

If he is wearing thick clothing, like thick denim jeans, you might find that grabbing the area is not as easy as you'd wish. But sometimes just going for that area can elicit a response and you can try something else at that time while he reacts with you going for the groin.

A final note. Hitting the groin, if done correctly, could be a very dangerous and life-changing thing to do to a man. If you're just annoyed with someone and he's not really a physical threat to you but you go ahead and hit him like I've told you then there might be serious consequences for that. I take violence quite seriously and I don't want to teach it for the use of people who might use it just because they got annoyed. If he is just annoying you then there are other channels you can take, like reporting him to the police or the workplace or to his family or friends. But if you're in a self defence situation, then you should use the necessary force to defend yourself, whatever level of force you can justify at the time.

THE NAVEL

The navel area is a good area to dig your elbows into if you're on the ground, to get a reaction, or even jab your thumb or jaw into. It is the area between the groin and bellybutton and is usually sensitive to being pressed strongly. I said to jab it because that is what appears to get the best reaction from it. A sudden sharp jab deep into the area, pushing deep, is likely to get a reaction. No way will it stop the fight for you, although I have winded someone badly enough when I punched him there as hard as I could during a 'no-rules' sparring session. I technically knocked him out because he was unable to move or do anything at all. So a good powerful shot there could help you but that takes practice and skill. But if that area presents itself, when you're on the floor or standing, then hit it really hard with one of the tools you're going to learn very soon (Palm Heels, elbows, headbutts or any tool you find).

THE FLOATING RIBS

These are the ribs at the very bottom of your ribcage. They're called floating because, unlike all the other ribs, these attach at the back of the spine but then do not attach at the front of the ribcage. That means they are 'floating'. And so they are quite weak in comparison to the rest of the ribcage. In fact the lower part of the ribcage, pretty much all round, at the front and at your sides, is all quite a lot weaker structurally than the rest of it and so for that reason this area is susceptible to big impacts. You also have the liver and stomach located about this area and hitting them can get some reactions, including stoppage if you deliver enough impact there with a hard shot or accumulated impact.

You can hit this area when standing up but a great time to remember to hit it is when you're on the ground. It really doesn't like being hit hard with anything like your knuckles or the heel of your foot or headbutts. It could make him react even if hit only reasonably hard, and a very powerful shot here could damage the area enough to cause quite severe pain.

However, this area might not be so easy to target if it's winter and Bad Guy is wearing a thick coat but in the summer it's fair game through thinner shirts.

THE SOLAR PLEXUS AND STERNUM

This area is not one place but on the body they lead on from one another, so often you can just aim for the general direction. To get real effect here you must generate strong impact forces. A good hit to the solar plexus is best delivered in secret. When he doesn't expect it it has much better consequences. It can basically stop him breathing for a few seconds as the wind is knocked out of him. The same applies to the sternum. I have, on a couple of occasions, hit people on the sternum and it made them lose breath and cough for a second or two as their lungs shook. Sometimes that's all you need to get away or to continue attacking with other shots. But this area does require hard hits to effect it usefully.

THE NECK

I'll cover this essential area later.

THE HEAD

You know to hit the head. I don't even need to tell you that. It's one of the main targets.

Remember that you can hit the head with your own body parts or with any object that you have.

You can also hit the head onto an object. So you can take the head and smack it into a wall or the floor etcetera. (Something I found out the hard way. I still have a hole at the side of my lip to remind me about it, where my incisor came through after my face met a toilet bowl in an unwelcome manner one day).

So we are talking about impact on the head. At this time. Hit it with a heavy object.

The Palm Heel is the master shot to hit the head with, but use whatever comes along at the time. Just because it's the best doesn't mean you can't get the job done with other shots. We're going to go over the Palm Heel, and more about the head, in a bit.

But you can hit the head with something sharp too. The end of a key will really hurt anywhere on the head and face, including the scalp. Stab it and scratch deep.

By 'the head' I mean the entire area above the neck. The whole area is susceptible to being hit and/or having sharp objects directed at it.

You can also shake the head violently and this can cause momentary dizziness/confusion. You need to grab the head with both hands and shake it as hard as you can to have that effect. It just allows you to take control of the situation while you're shaking and for him to lose control of himself at that time. As soon as you stop though he regains control almost immediately. (This is actually a technique that works very well against someone wearing a bike helmet, whether motorbike or bicycle. You can grab it and shake, and twist it about, then drag them to the ground or push them away. But these are ninja assassin techniques we are heading into now. Let's get back to the bread and butter, the high percentage techniques that are needed more often).

So, as you can see, we can make the head quite a lot more vulnerable than you probably realised. There's more to come later about it!

THE EYES. THE NOSE. THE EARS

To start with these are all poke-able, with your fingers or a key or a pen or the end of your comb or brush. You do want to poke very deep though. If you're squeamish then don't listen to this bit: but if the situation is serious you need to poke right into the back of his eye. Not a surface poke as it will have very little effect at stopping him. But for less intense situations you might only need to strongly tap the eye and that's enough to get someone to back off.

With the nose it doesn't like being squished flat to the face. It doesn't like a something being inside and then pulling the nostrils and it doesn't like something going deep up it either. What it doesn't like is what you'll need to do if you're in need to saving yourself.

With the ears you can cup your hand and whack it over the ear to create a kind of pressure in his ear. It probably won't burst his eardrum and at best might cause him to get dizzy. But just a good strike of any kind to the ear is going to make some ringing sounds and make birds fly around his head for a second.

Hit the ear with anything hard. You can poke your index finger or thumb (or a pen or keys) in there and drive it in hard too. It's just unpleasant. He should react, in which case he will move away from the pain.

If he's on the floor you can knee any of these areas or elbow them. You can Palm Heel them and use many of the other tools too.

NOTE. Just a reminder that for any of the targets, whether you use your own body parts to attack or you use an object you have adapted as a weapon to help you, you will need to go hard and you will need to repeat the action until you have the result you want. If things are serious then that is what you will have to do if you want to get out.

Now that you know where to hit him, let's have a look at some of the best tools you can use to do that with!

HOW TO HURT HIM:
THE TOOLS YOU NEED

Firstly you must understand the purpose of hitting him. Why are you hitting him?

The main purpose is to get him to stop what he is doing to you.

This could be something less serious expanding all the way up to very serious.

You could also hit him to distract him.

Maybe so he loosens his grip and you can escape. Maybe to make him think about you hitting him when actually you're going to bite him. And so on.

Deception and distraction are great additions to your tactical toolbox and really do enhance much of what you do. Trick him whenever you can. It's a game he's playing with you. Play it back, but better.

To make him stop or to distract him when you hit him he actually needs to notice that you hit him. So your shot has to have an effect. In other words, if you hit him harder, he's more likely to realise he's been hit. If you hit him hard enough, and enough times, you might stop him.

We're going to learn what tools you can hit him with. Again, as you've probably realised by now, since it's a running theme through this book, you know most of these but my job is to make them better for you. My role is to help you enhance your natural abilities and knowledge.

Later, during your second read of this book, you can add The Magic Five to these shots to make them twice, five times, maybe ten times more powerful. The Magic Five will be in Part Four and really do take things to a whole other level.

Note that it often doesn't matter what you hit him with. Just hit with the tool that is most available at the time. Some tools will distract and disrupt him more than others though but we can't always choose what we are going to hit with. We hit with what is available to us at the time and we hit the target that is available to us at the time.

Just as an example, let's say your favourite go-to shot is the punch. You want to punch him but he's grabbed you and his head is below your head. You can only hit the top of his head. You're now unable to punch because punching the top of his head is going to hurt you more than him. The punch has been neutralised.

But you still have other tools available - for example downwards elbows, or hammer-fists or Palm Heels. All three tools are available to do the job. You might use one but you might use all three, one after the other.

So, although you maybe favour one shot, it is not always available to you.

Just to let you know from the off - the Palm Heel strike is the single most useful tool and is available in far more places than anything else. It is also the most powerful shot there is if you develop it, especially using The Magic Five. I recommend you always practice the Palm Peel and practice it from every position and make it the go-to in your toolbox.

One more thing about learning strikes (strike/striking is the martial art word for hitting). There are ten thousand different ways you can hit someone. Spinning backfists, flying kicks, superman punches. These are all really fancy, look great when used by Marvel Superheroes and sometimes by martial artists, who are showing their skills and athletic abilities. But these shots have very specific and rare uses. What we want are the simple things that work powerfully, work often and work almost everywhere. Moves that are universally applicable, remember? Moves we can use when standing, kneeling or on the floor. Moves that can be used in a confined space like a car or a hotel room and can also be used in open spaces. Universal application as much as we can.

So here are the most useful shots and the reality of using them.

PUNCHES

Let's begin with the punch. The go-to for most people who hit you and probably your go-to as well at this time.

Everyone roughly knows how to punch. You make a fist and deliver the knuckles into the object you want to hurt. You hit with the knuckles, whilst keeping your wrist locked tight and aligned.

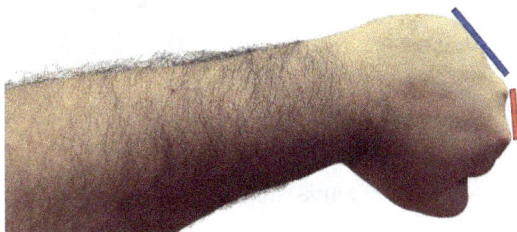

Some people punch with the three smaller knuckles (blue line). Others punch with the two big ones (red line, as shown).

Note (below) how the blue arrow shows the fist to be in a straight line with the wrist. This should generally be the case but more important than alignment is to keep this area solid, even if it is a little bent. Otherwise you will damage your wrist and it's very painful too. I say this from experience.

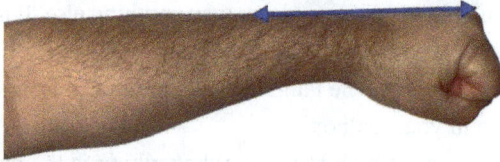

Here's the reality of punching, and a quick tip.

The reality is that when you hit someone's big head, hit them anywhere on the scull or jaw or even the cheek bones, with your much smaller hands, you're very likely to injure yourself. Men hitting men will regularly hurt their knuckles after just a single punch. They will often break a hand after a punch. At the very least, punching the head with non-gloved hands is very painful.

A trained boxer who's been punching bags and faces for eternity will actually have hands conditioned like concrete. This is due to Wolff's Law, which says minutely broken bones will heal to the strength of concrete over a long period of time. That's why boxers have hands literally like concrete and Thai boxers have shins of steel. But I know that most boxers have at least one damaged hand due to years of hitting things even though their hands were bandaged most of the time.

Beyond a boxer's concrete hands, anyone who punches without some nice wrapping and gloves over their knuckles, will break their hands very quickly and painfully.

If you watch any of the old no-holds barred fighting, where they didn't wear gloves, you'll see these men - who were professional fighters - rarely punching. They slapped - or in the case of Bas Rutten he used palm heels to become a no-rules competitive fighting superstar.

If you punch hard, expect to break your hands. It's that simple.

But does that mean you should never punch in a live situation? No, that's not the point. The point is that you need to be aware that punching can damage your hands and this will hurt a lot when it does. So be aware that there are better shots most of the time. (Have I mentioned the Palm Heel yet?!)

So where is the punch most effective? When you're hitting softer targets. So hitting the jaw might be okay if you're not hitting it full on (and preferably hitting it at an angle). Punching into the eyes could have an effect. Hitting the nose.

Hitting the floating ribs. Hitting the testicles. Hitting into the kidneys or liver. Hitting the ear. Hitting the neck. Hitting the back of the neck.

You can hit accumulated punches rather than one super hard shot in some positions too.

There are many places and times you want to punch. If you choose to punch the face and head at your full capacity, then that's your choice. I just think that for most of you it will not have the effect you imagine it will, so please be ready for that.

However, it might buy you a second to run away though. It might buy you a second to break free from something.

The punch is a very nuanced thing and I just wanted to make sure you understood it in the grand scheme of things when it comes to self defence.

So if you do punch, like with all strikes that you do, be ready to use the next moment to do something else too.

One shot on its own rarely works anyway, whether it's a punch or anything else.

KNEES AND KICKS

Another major go-to for most women is the knee or kick to the groin. We've covered the kicking to the groin already (using a snap-kick) and if you were to do it with your knees then the process is similar. Drive your knee upwards, connect with his groin, and make sure you continue using your upwards momentum to keep driving, so he is taken off the ground, flies in the air for a bit. That's what you want to be trying to do. It is a metaphor. It is very unlikely you will be able to lift him off the floor. But, please, do try.

When you knee someone it actually isn't the 'knee' you hit them with. It's not the kneecap. It is the area just above that. I'd say technically you are hitting them with the lowest part of your thigh rather than the knee itself. I just wanted to ensure you knew that so you can really get it right and drive that knee right up to the heavens.

With regards kicks. The general consensus in the martial arts is that the Muay Thai roundhouse kick is the king of them all. I agree with that since it has proven itself for a very long time and in every fighting arena.

Here's the issue with it - it is a very technical move and takes a lot of practice to get right. It's also not so easy to use if your footwear isn't right or you're on slippery or uneven ground. I've been lucky enough to have trained with a couple of world Muay Thai champions and I know the ins and outs of the roundhouse better than most but I keep it back as a move used in sparring rather than as a first shot in self defence. I have it as a tool that's ready to use but that's because I've got a lot of other tools that I've sharpened over the years so I can afford to keep this one in my weaponry.

(Can you guess what my first shot would be in pretty much every given situation? I bet you can figure it out now! Though I shouldn't have told you that. Once word gets out, any time I need to defend myself, the attacker will know that I'm going to start with a Palm Heel. Oh well.)

We're not going to learn the Muay Thai roundhouse here. It's too much and there's so many variations of it but feel free to Google it and have a go, or ask me to teach it to you, though it will take some time.

The next best kick after the Muay Thai roundhouse is the push-kick. It is probably the second most used move in Muay Thai but is also a staple of many kickboxing arts and often used in the cage fights of modern Mixed Martial Arts.

Here's what it looks like.

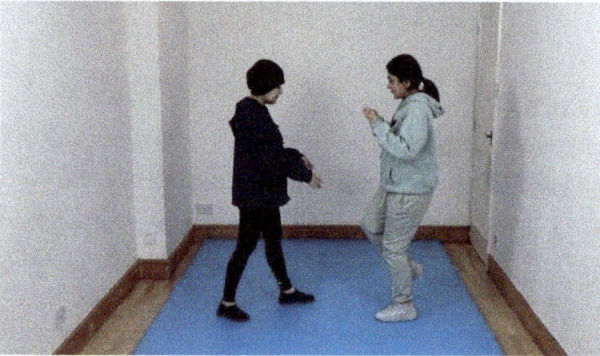

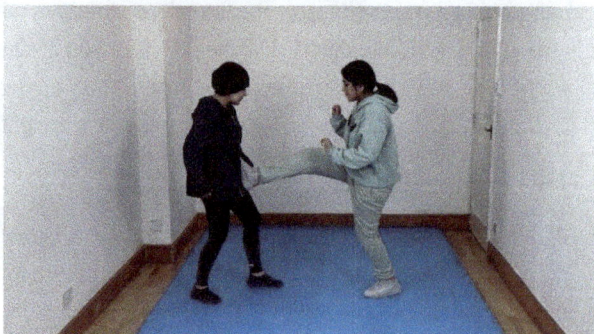

There are some things to note with the push-kick.

Firstly, your foot will land (on the attacker's stomach/navel most likely) where they can potentially grab it. This is actually a natural instinct and they will do it without thinking. So be ready to deal with having your leg grabbed if you do a push-kick. You'll need to probably hit them in the face (palm heel/punch) to get them to release your grabbed leg. Personally, I use the push-kick but in a sharp jabbing kind of motion. It was the first kick I ever learned, back in karate when I was a kid. It does work. I've seen people hit solid brick walls using this kick, for training purposes, and seen the walls come apart over time. But it does require some practice to get it right regularly.

ELBOWS
Another favourite for women is using the elbows. There are many ways to use elbows in striking. It could be a short book in itself.

They are devastating when used correctly, and even more so when you add The Magic Five to them.

The area you want to use when employing elbows is anywhere from about halfway along your forearm all the way to the elbow bone itself. You want any part of this - or most of it - to connect with him. With force.

If you elbow him, just remember to try to hit vulnerable parts like the eyeball or nose or across the temple or groin or across the neck or ears. For you, those are the places you can really have effect.

The one great thing about elbows is that you can elbow in pretty much any direction- up/down/left/right/forwards and even backwards at someone behind you. Have a think about that and have a go at it.

For more on elbow strikes and a complete foundation-level training, have a look at our course One Step Ahead and get one step ahead of the attacker. www.power-for-women.org/onestepahead.

YOUR HEAD IS A BUTT
I'm so sorry. Your head is not a butt really! I only said that because I'm childish and I wanted to get your attention. But…the headbutt is a dangerous tool.

Be aware that it can be used against you, just like any of the other shots we talk about here, though the headbutt is very rare and only used by real thugs who've got a lot of experience at being thugs. More 'civilised' people are less likely to use it.

And that's where there is the advantage for you! It would be quite unexpected for a woman to use it in any situation, whether standing or on the ground, but especially on the ground.

The headbutt really is a very vicious tool and can stop an attack quickly if it lands correctly. Headbutts are most effective when you sneak them in. They can be used from pretty much any distance and any position on the floor if you're on top of him.

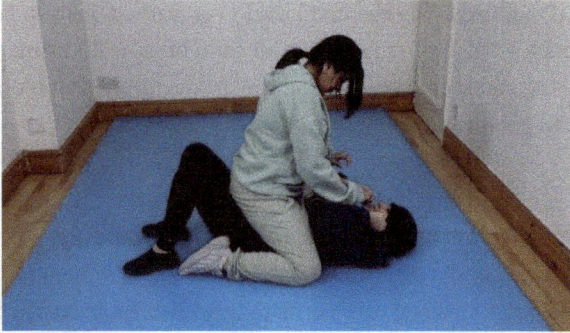

You might be here sitting upright on top in the Full Mount for example.

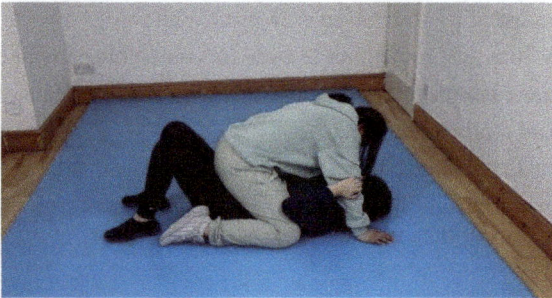

Or being pulled down.

Both these places you just have to drop your head quickly into him several times to make him release you.

To make the headbutt effective you need to hit using only the area above your eyebrows and you hit him only on the area below the eyebrows. Read that again, please. Do not clash your scull into his scull. It's going to really hurt you. Hit him with your forehead or top of your head or back of your head and hit him all across the face and ears and jaw and neck.

Here in the Cross-Side position you can turn towards him and headbutt (repeatedly) at the face and neck and ears.

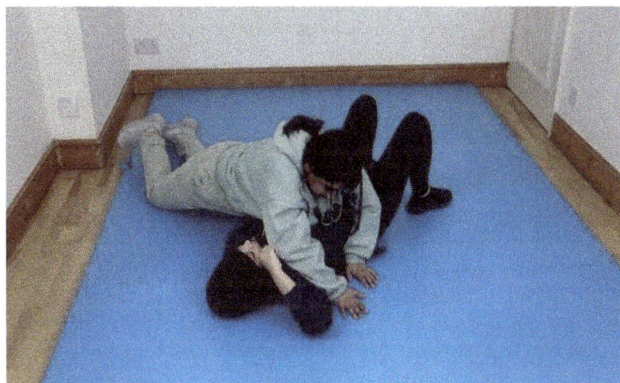

If you are being pulled downwards like this…

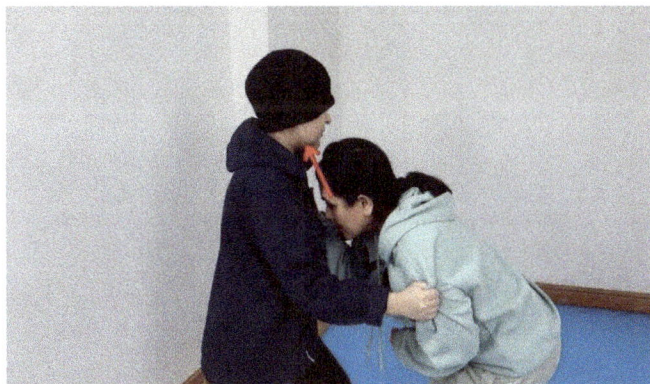

You could easily drive/jump your head upwards and hit his chin with your scull. This can be quite an effective move if someone is trying to push you down or drag you away.

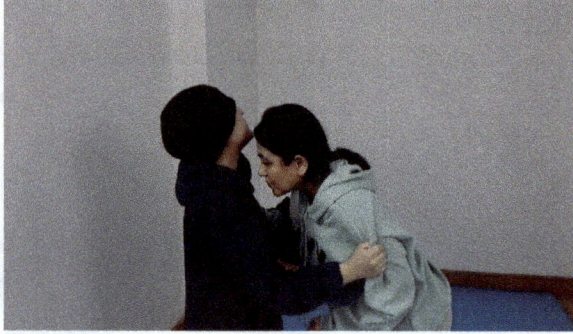

As their head lifts up, you can headbutt their face in a forwards motion to follow up what you've already done.

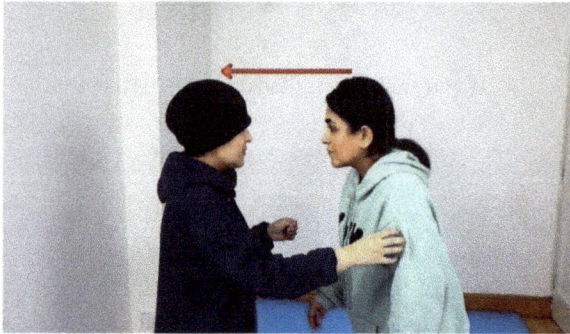

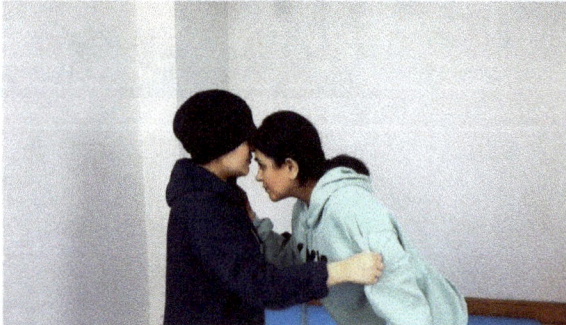

Obviously you can use the forwards headbutt at other times too, for example if he's trying to pull you forwards to take you away you might be able to drive it at his face.

The headbutt works very well on the face but it can also be used to strike the sternum, the floating ribs, the groin, the navel and even the side of his neck too. You can use it in other ways too if you think about it, so it is quite an effective move, but one that women seem to shy away from for some reason.

PRACTISING HEADBUTTS

When you learn and/or practice headbutts, do not go full-out. Practice the technique very lightly at all times. Don't knock yourself out on a punch-bag or something else, please.

You can hit with the back of your scull too if he is behind you, whether you are standing up or on the floor.

For women, I think the headbutt is a most useful tool and one you can use quite easily, so do add it to your armoury.

A NOTE ABOUT HITTING HIM (before we move on to the Palm Heel. Yippee!!)

You can hit him with any part of your body really.

We haven't covered all the ways to hit someone but covered all the most useful ones you could use (and practice) right now.

You can hit him with items you're carrying or items in your bag.

I've seen mobile phone corners used to jab someone in the eye or used to hit the back of the hand or into the face. It is a metal object after all. It can be used in other ways too, to break fingers and suchlike, which are out of the scope of this book.

Remember you can use strikes to send him away from you. You can punch or kick him into the road or canal or off the edge of the balcony of a hotel room.

So don't forget to power through with your shot. Get as much of your energy transferred into him as you possibly can.

Nice.

Let's finally move on to the Palm Heel.

THE ONE SHOT
THAT RULES THEM ALL

The Palm Heel is a disputed empress of the martial arts but she's disputed only by those who specialise in one area only. So the boxer says the punch is superior because that's what he or she specialises in. The kickboxer will say the roundhouse kick is the most effective tool, or the push-kick. The wrestler will say that the throw is better than the punch. And so on it goes. Each has their favourite.

I also have a favourite - the punch is my favourite shot. It is the one I learned first. It is the one I have practised most in my life. It is my baby that has helped me so many time. It is visceral and it feels good when you connect with a Bad Guy. But it is at best the King of the strikes. I am fully aware of that.

The Palm Heel is the real ruler of all.

I'm not saying the others are useless. They are certainly not. It's just for self defence purposes, you should spend a lot of time on the Palm Heel and really know it.

It should be the first strike you learn if you're a beginner. It should be the first one you teach your daughter (or son). It should be the first one you always consider whether you're standing or on the ground. You can use it almost everywhere.

Whether the person is taller than you or shorter doesn't matter to the Palm Heel. It's got a job to do and it's going to do it.

If someone is ducking down (maybe to get at your legs), or someone has turned away from you and is presenting the side or back of their head; the Palm Heel will do its job.

You can use the palm heel if someone is lying on top of you. You can use it when you're on top of someone else.

You can use it if someone is between your legs when you're on the floor. You can use it out to the sides rather that straight in front of you.

It is the single most effective strike there is.

I know I'm going on about it (or the ADHD is) but I just want to make sure you know my feelings on this.

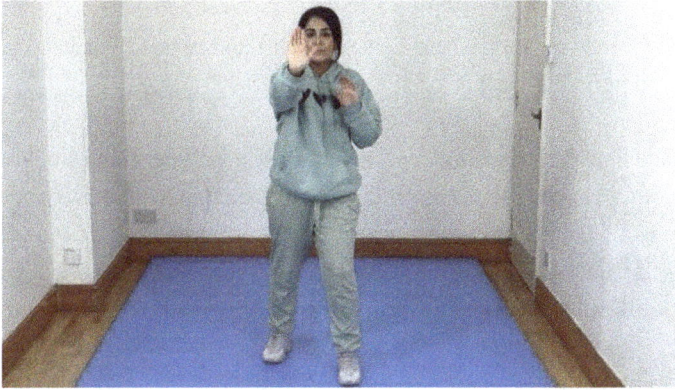

You can use the Palm heel if you're on your way down to the ground. Or whilst you're getting back up. You can use it if you're kneeling or sitting. You can use it if you're in a car or in a train carriage. You can use it under water (Yes, of course there's a martial art covering underwater fighting! It's part of the Russian Systema artform that their military special forces claim to use).

This next bit will be debated by martial artists…but in my experience you can also generate more power with a Palm Heel than a punch in most positions.

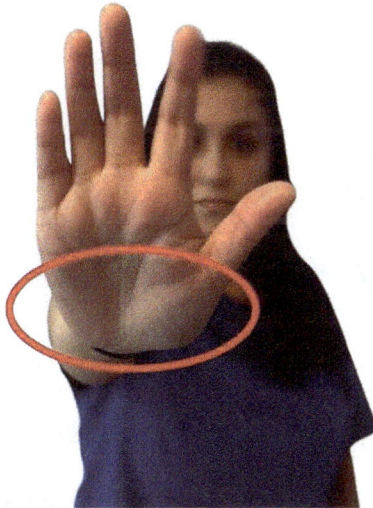

If you doubt me then ask Bas Rutten who loves Palm Heel shots and says it is the most powerful shot when bare knuckled. He should know.

So when you do a Palm Heel strike you need to hit them with the area of the hand that is circled in the above photo.

You need to pull your fingers back too when you do it and be careful not to get them caught in the clothing of the Bad Guy.

Keep your hand somewhere between solid and relaxed but keep your wrist rigid as you pull your fingers back.

Sounds like a lot of instruction but basically keep your fingers out of the way so they don't get caught in something. Other than that just hit away.

Here is the Palm Heel being used in various different positions so you can see for yourself. Have a go with your partner or just 'shadow box' these in your living room or workplace bathroom when you can get away from the computer.

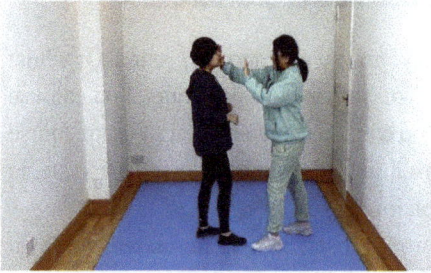

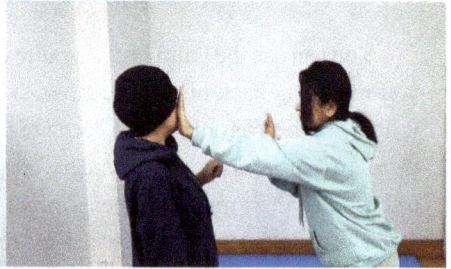

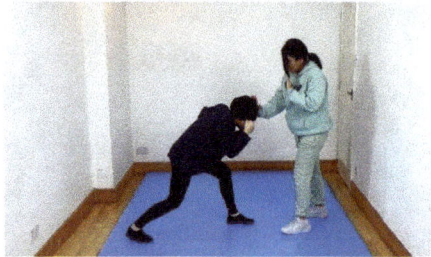

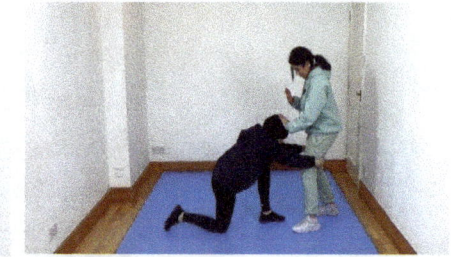

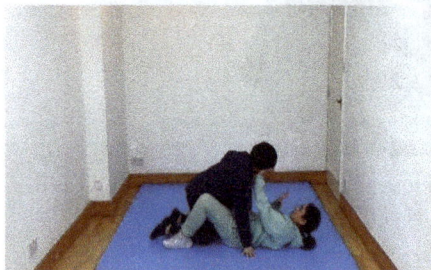

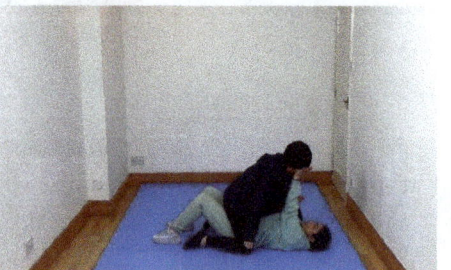

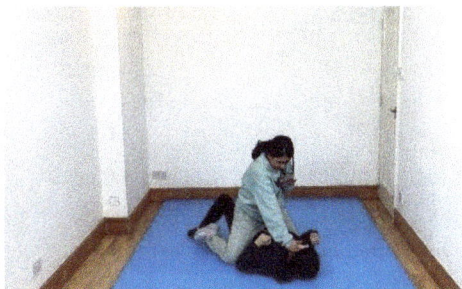
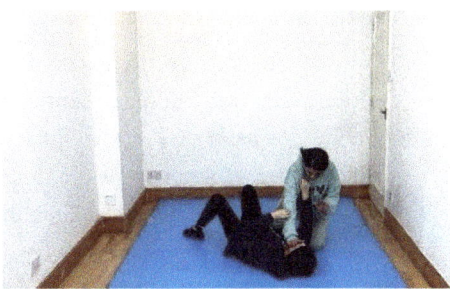

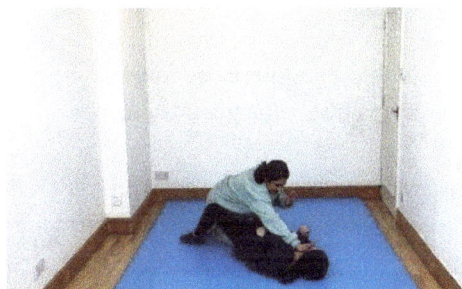
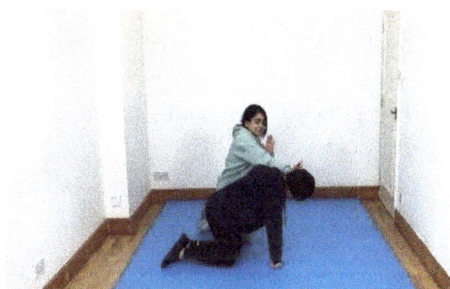

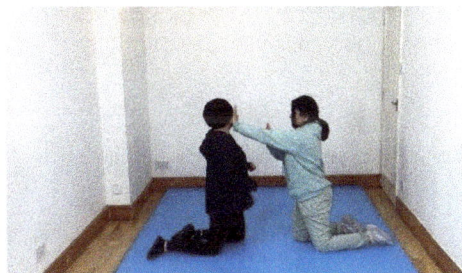
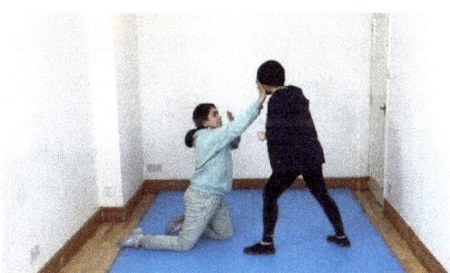

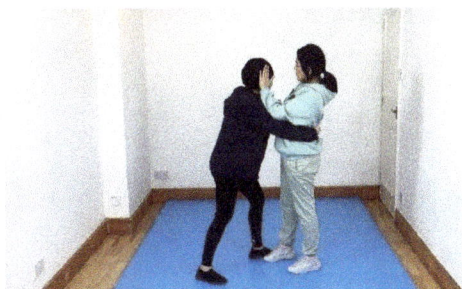
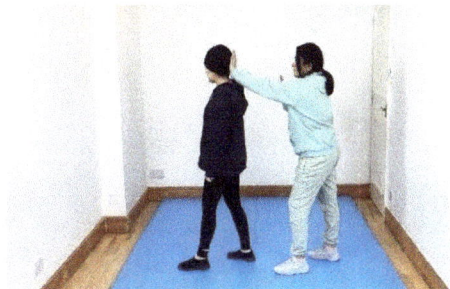

It is an amazing shot for the head and face and neck. Even if there is a hand in the way of the Palm Heel you can often still hit right through.

Remember that you're not confined to just the head area. You can hit the groin too. For example, if you're kneeling.

In practice, if you can slam a door shut (and I know ALL of you can!) then you can Palm Heel. It is almost the same action. In fact, if no one is watching, go and slam a door several times. Drive your whole bodyweight into it so it really slams. Just make sure your boss isn't behind it, or your mum isn't home or you're not doing it in the university library during the busy period. (You have to be quiet in libraries apparently and you're not allowed to slam doors in the boss's face either. Rules, eh. Who needs 'em?).

Genuinely, the action of slamming a door shut is almost the same as doing a Palm Heel. If you can't get to a door, just imagine yourself doing it and practice in your head.

Slam that door shut really really hard. Put your weight and body behind your movement.

Whatever it takes, even if you have to break many doors, learn the Palm Heel.

(Please note that I don't actually want you to slam doors and break them. But you get the idea that the action for Palm Heeling is pretty much the same as doing that. I hope you haven't damaged anything).

You can add even more power to the Palm Heel (and any other strike or push or pull for that matter when you add The Magic Five, so do come back and have a go at it when you've learned about them).

OH, WHAT A PAIN!

We have mentioned pain already but it's worthy of having its own short chapter. It's often believed by those who have never been in a deeply dangerous confrontation that pain will stop an attacker.

The fact is that the only things that guarantees you will not be attacked further is a stoppage - unconsciousness and beyond. And that is it. We are talking about serious situations here, life threatening ones. Up until he is unconscious or deceased, he might not stop. I've seen a man with a broken arm - broken at the elbow during the fight - trying to hit his nemesis by swinging the broken and non-functioning arm, trying to use it as a club to whack him with! An actual arm completely broken.

Some people will succumb to pain while others revel in it. Some are tolerant more than others. Some can ignore it. Some will be on drugs or drink and not feel a thing. (The majority of attacks on women have alcohol consumption involved to some level). Decades spent in training, fighting, competing and in police work has taught me a lot about physical pain. Pain in others as well as myself. I have a very high tolerance to pain when I'm motivated or angered. Aren't you the same?

I've crossed paths with others who can tolerate plenty of pain. Here's one example I saw with my own eyes.

A Bad Guy was shot with two police tasers at the same time. Unimaginable pain for most of us. Tasers really hurt.

This only stopped him for the couple of seconds the taser was first applied before he cut the wires with the two chef's knives he was carrying. Moments before he had been running through the streets and had actually knocked on random houses and asked to be let in whilst he held the knives in his hands. This was at 2am.

You can see why he was tasered.

But he had bypassed the immense pain and managed to cut the TWO taser wires that were pumping the pain into his body.

He swung the machetes like a madman and chased the officers. Being British police officers and not wanting to spend three days writing paperwork and a month on suspended duties they first ran away rather than shoot him with real bullets. But he forced them to take action and they shot him five times. Bear in mind that this was in the U.K. and that meant that each shot was deliberated, cogitated and considered before the trigger was pulled so it probably took a few seconds to discharge the five rounds. He did not stop his attack until the fifth bullet went into him.

The point is that pain from each individual bullet didn't send enough signals to his brain to stop his attack.

And bullets are famous for being painful and being able to stop most people.

Another exceptional occasion I have to mention is when I saw a man, with really severe face and neck injuries, actually argue with police officers who were trying to save his life. I won't describe too much but he had head-butted the passenger side window of a car and then not pulled his head back out in a safe way.

He'd not been careful to say the least. It was one of the worst injuries I've ever seen and it actually made me squirm looking at it and it's even making me squirm thinking about it right now.

He was about to bleed to death if he didn't let officers help him right away but he was arguing with them, fearing he was about to be arrested for what he'd done. So they forced him to the ground to treat him but even with those severe injuries he was fighting them off. Once officers had secured him and somehow managed to stem the bleeding and kept him alive, as they walked him to the ambulance he was still arguing with them whilst they held bandages to his neck and face. He was later found to have taken cocaine and had been drinking most of the day. He did live in the end, in case you're wondering but I have no idea how.

Neither of these two men showed any signs of pain distress and both were happy to go on fighting.

Oh, by the way, the machete guy was also high on cocaine and I genuinely don't know if he lived or died because I was already onto my next job within an hour of that happening. That's London for you on some nights.

I've got more stories like these. Every police officer and soldier has and they'll tell you about pain - tolerant attackers because it's really not all that uncommon.

Some women choose to give birth without painkillers! Let's not forget that either! They can mentally work their way through hours and hours of what many consider is the most painful thing there is.

We have to agree that pain is something we cannot fully rely on to help us stop an attacker. It's a good tool to think about and keep in our arsenal because it will work in some of the lesser serious instances. But we can also say that it can fail to stop him if he's fired up on adrenaline, excitement, alcohol or drugs and commitment.

I don't want that to be your final takeaway about using pain though. I just wanted to make sure you knew that it can fail so that at that time you're not left with a broken mind that's wondering what's going on. You'll have enough to do in a self defence situation as it is. If we can remove many of the surprises we can stay a step ahead of the situation and so you need to be aware of this.

Pain does work in the majority of cases, when the intent of the attacker can be broken. When he can be deterred. When he knows you're going to fight back. In those cases it might be enough to put him off and you can get away.

It also can be used as a tactic to get a reaction from him, so he moves his hands away, allowing you to get to a more vulnerable part of him. Or it could be used to break his grip etcetera.

And in many cases, those that are not too serious, those which are actually the more common, it is often enough to deter him from continuing his actions.

So do use pain, but remember that in the context of a serious self defence situation, it might not stop him. To guarantee stopping him, in those rare situations where your mental or physical life is in real danger, you have to use more severe skills that will make him unconscious or even send him back to meet his Maker.

But if he's forced you there, you can't be blamed if that's the only option he's left you to take.

"TO BREATHE OR NOT TO BREATHE?"
THAT IS THE QUESTION

So that's a silly question and I put it that way to get your attention in the hope you'll notice and remember this info below if sh%t happens.

Of course you need to breathe!

But there are a few things you need to understand about breathing when it comes to being in a physical altercation.

The single most important thing to know is that you are very likely to 'get out of breath' in some kind of way. The most vicious of these is if you get winded, when you get the 'breath knocked out' of you. You can get winded if you are hit hard or if you fall.

When your breath is knocked out, it means you can't breath in or out. The diaphragm and intercostals stop and your stomach and entire body clenches up so tight it feels like your soul is leaving your body. It's quite painful, in other words, and when it's happened to me (too many times) I felt as if I couldn't get my lungs to breath again. That's how it feels. It is a terrible feeling. As if your breathing apparatus has just switched off and you cannot switch them back on.

It usually takes a very long few seconds to recover and you'll often be doubled over at the waist, holding that area to comfort it.

It often occurs after a hit to the solar plexus or any part of the breathing apparatus, including the ribs. I've had it happen in sparring when someone hit me square across the sternum and it felt as if my lungs just stopped. I recognised it as the same effect as when you are thrown to the ground and don't manage to breakfall. On another occasion I was kicked full-on into the side of my ribs and again I was in a similar position. This time I believe my rib muscles (the intercostals) had been shocked and they stopped functioning for a while. You can't breathe easily if your ribs can't move to let the lungs expand.

So you need to be aware of these things so they're a bit less of a shock should they happen to you during an altercation.

You haven't died and you're very unlikely to. Just hang in there, and 'relax' as much as you can so the system starts to work again. Did I just tell you to relax when someone has just hit you? I know it might not be as easy as that but it will take a few seconds to recover from being winded. You just have to wait it out if that's all you can do. The good thing is that you will recover from being winded very quickly and with no side effects. So that is something to note and look forward to.

Of course, if there is damage to the area then that is another matter. I am only talking about being winded here.

Another way you might lose your breath is through excessive exertion. If you try too hard, more than your aerobic system can handle, then you'll be out of breath and rapidly lose power.

Adrenaline affects your breath so you'll have at least some kind of breathing difference to consider from the start.

So all these things could affect your breathing when you fight. They're not going to be pleasant to deal with! But knowing about them takes a small bit of the shock away if it happens to you.

So is there a way to deal with this lack of energy or when you get out of breath through over-exertion?

What fighters do to relieve pain and to energise themselves or to push through difficult bits of a fight is the 'suck it up'. That's what fighters and coaches call it. This is in reference to sucking up the air. So what they do is take big deep breaths. They do this on purpose rather than letting their body decide when to breathe. They take conscious control of their breathing, and they take a big deep breath in and then let it out, and repeat.

Have a quick go at this right now if it is safe for you to do so, and you are medically cleared to do so.

Basically breathe in really deep. It can be from your mouth or nose. As you breathe in make sure your rib cage is allowed to extend forwards, upwards and to the sides. The back of the ribcage should be allowed to extend backwards too. Expand the ribcage like it is a balloon. You need to also let your belly relax and get big like a balloon too. Push you bellybutton outwards. This is actually more important than anything else - getting your belly full.

That's the in-breath.

Once your lungs are full, relax as much as you can and let the breath out. You can push it out if you want but a long relaxed emptying takes more carbon dioxide out.

If your out breath is longer than the in-breath you will absorb more oxygen and eliminate more unusable carbon dioxide.

Repeat this a few times.

Now, if you are in a physical altercation (or even if you're struggling with weights or cardio in the gym) this is the breathing technique you should use.

This is practically the 'diaphragmatic breathing technique' you might have heard of. This also affects the Vargas nerve, which is a very good thing for you (read up about it. I can't be making this book any longer than it is already!).

You could include diaphragmatic breathing into your daily life if you wanted to. It has a tonne of benefits.

But for the time you need to protect yourself, it is a vital type of breathing, and one employed by many professional fighters when the going gets tough.

One more thing I should mention about breathing during a self defence situation is that you won't notice it or think about it until you're actually out of breath. That's when your brain will push you to take notice. Prior to that there is enough going on for you to deal with and it's unlikely you'll be thinking about your breath.

But the key thing is that when you first notice your breathing, whether it's before any confrontation even starts or anytime during it, or even as you run away, then it's time to take control of that breath for yourself and get some deep belly breaths done. At the very least it will affect the Vargus nerve, and I've already said that's a very good thing.

HE'S GRABBING YOU

So in Stage Three you are now dealing with someone who's begun attacking you. It could be that this person has talked to you first, tricked you or diverted your attention, bypassed your natural protective instincts, and then attacked.

Maybe you were in The Fence but he's got past your Fence and attacked you.

Or maybe it was all too quick and you didn't even raise an arm nevermind the full Fence.

As the situation gets physical there are only a few things that can happen.

From his point of view, these are the only three things he can do.

He can hit you or he can grab you or he can combine both of those. That's it.

Of course there are many variables to each of those, but doesn't it make it a little clearer to know that there are only two/three things he can actually do?

So let's first deal with him grabbing you.

To understand how to deal with being grabbed we must first understand where we might be grabbed.

So, this could be **limbs**, **clothes**, around the **torso** (usually called a 'bear hug') and **hair**.

That's it. He might switch between these areas, and he might switch between holding us with one hand or two, but that's it.

So let's expand on these a little prior to discovering ways to avoid and/or escape the early grabs.

The limbs - the most likely thing is to have your arms grabbed at the wrists, forearms, elbows, or even at the bicep/tricep area. Anywhere really, but the wrist is usually the most common followed by forearms.

You could get your legs grabbed but that is more the case when you are on the floor. Clothes - this could be anywhere but the most likely areas are at the wrists, arms, shoulders and the lapel.

Body - he could grab your entire torso in a 'bear hug' from the front or the rear. He could also grab at your neck as in the headlock throw we have already shown.

Hair - he might take a full grab with his fingers deeply entangled with your hair. And that's about it.

As with most things in self defence, we want to do things as soon as possible.

If he's coming in for a grab, we want to knock his hands out of the way immediately. This works.

As soon as you see a hand coming to grab you, use your hand (shaped into a cupped palm) to whack his hand away instantly!

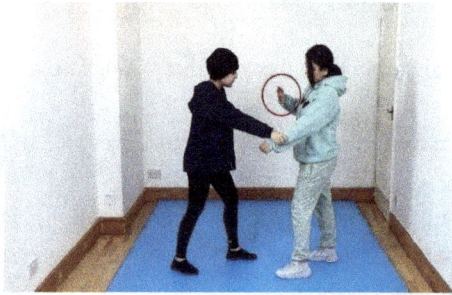

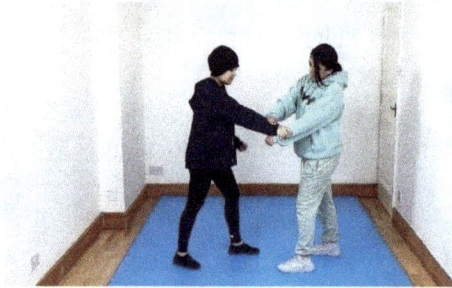

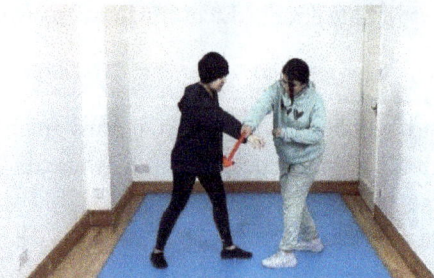

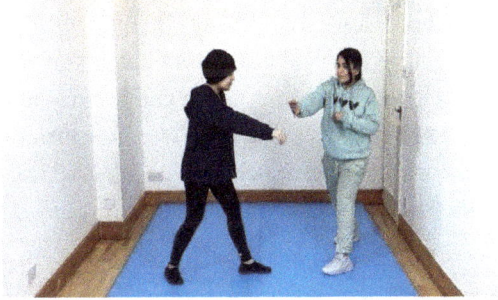

Then move away, keeping the Fence as you continue increasing the distance between you.

Let's say he's got past that stage and has grabbed something properly.

It takes a second or two for him to properly secure a hold.

So it's still possible to whack his hand off as shown above if you do it within this time, before he's secured the grip.

You can whack his hand directly or his arm at the elbow or biceps to complete the same technique.

So let's say you didn't whack his hands off early, didn't do it as soon as he grabbed you and now he's secured the grab.

Why are you being grabbed? It is one of two things. Either to move you somewhere or to control you where you are.

That's it. There is no other reason to grab you.

If he hits you, it's usually to subdue you to get better control or he hits you to distract you so you're focusing on the pain and damage while he drags or pushes you.

So, as you know, grabbing you is quite a serious situation and quite a scary one too.

If you get the chance, drop into the Wide Fence as you'll be able to resist him better. And, as usual, you have a direct defence to what he is doing (directly targeting any of the aspects of the grab) or indirectly dealing with it.

The most effective direct defences to the grab are quite easy when you know how but they work better as a system rather than just on their own. You need to be able to shake the person off in many ways because of the number of different ways you can be grabbed. However, it's quite simple when you know how. At Power for Women we have a course that covers this if you want to go that way. It's a whole system to break away from being grabbed. (Actually it starts with a man following you and how to deal with that. We show the Fence etc). But let's see what we can do about it in a book since we are here right now.

If you have your Fence up and he reaches forwards, he is likely to grab your arm this way.

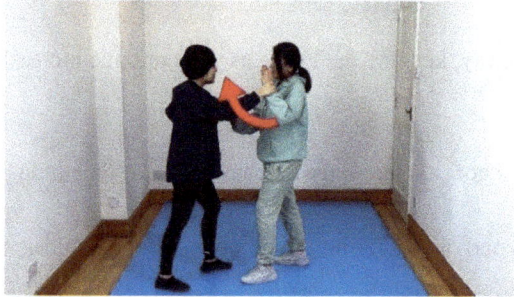

It is actually still quite possible to whack his arm off like before. Or you can get a little more technical and throw your elbow over the top like this.

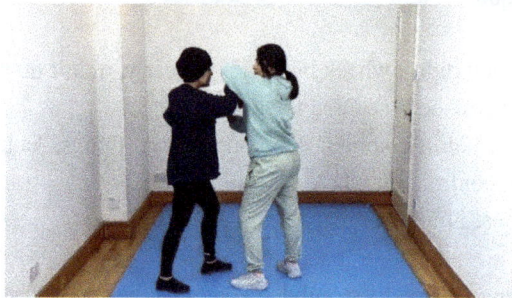

Remember that you are working against his wrist. The aim of the elbow is to apply pressure to the area he is holding you with, his hand in other words.

If he is holding both your arms like below, then you do one elbow and then the other. You cannot do both at the same time.

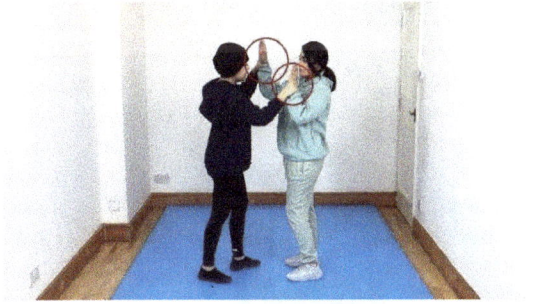

If he has grabbed your clothes at the wrist or arms you can use the same escape but if he grabs at your collar or lapel then there is slightly different way of doing things.

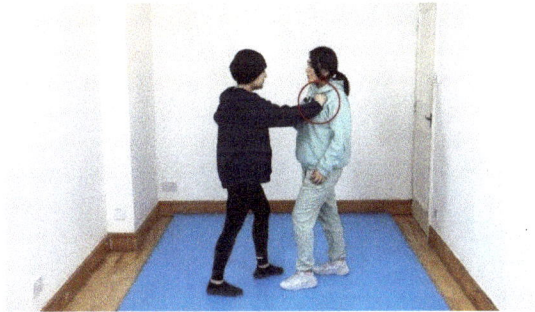

Above he has grabbed you at the collar.
This time you quickly cup both your hands like this…

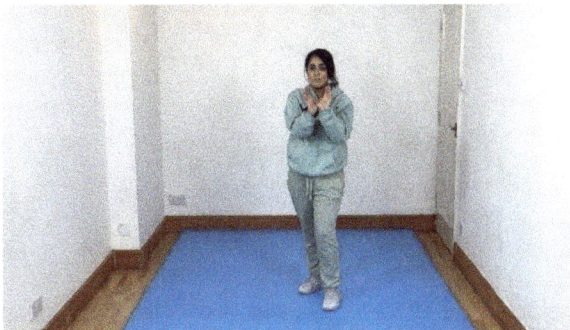

And drive them up to take his grip off, like this…

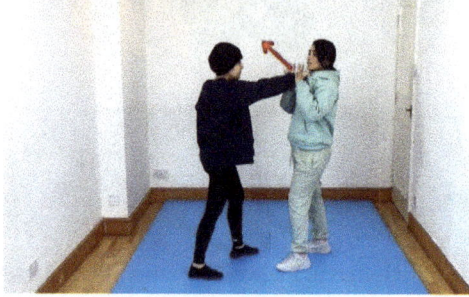

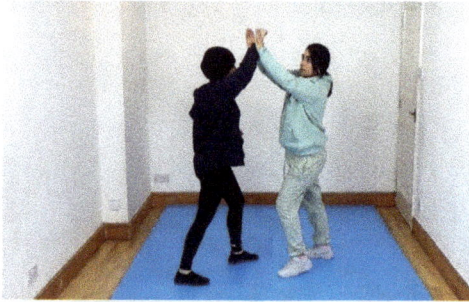

And make sure you are moving away as you let go of him. Get yourself back into The Fence too.

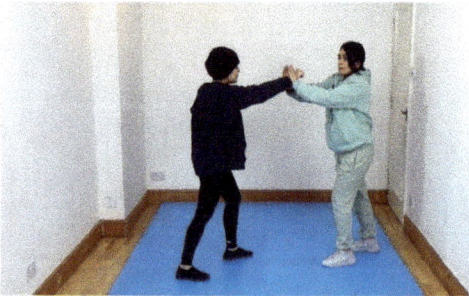

These moves are super effective and work really well even against trained judo and jiu jitsu fighters, who have the strongest grips in the martial arts and know you're going to do this them. Even they cannot hold on. That's how effective these moves are when done correctly.

They work whether he's holding your wrists or clothes. They work if he's holding one of your arms or both. They are very simple but very effective and are really worth knowing and practising because they can stop an altercation from progressing from the very start.

With your training partner you should have a go at these escapes. Get them to hold onto your lapel or onto your sleeve, then cup your free hand and whack their arm off.

Also try the elbow escapes. Get them to hold your arms and use your elbows to apply pressure to their fingers so they have to let go. Start gently to begin with. Learn the method. Then build up to doing it quickly and shaking them off as soon as you're grabbed.

Remember that if you've got both your arms being held then you need to do one elbow at a time.

You could also have a go attacking his fingers (as shown in the Bear Grabs chapter, next). Bend them or break them. You'll need to yank at one or two, twist them and use good strength to get them off. Going for the fingers is always a reliable go-to and it's not too easy to stop either as long as you are reasonably rapid at getting to it. Just make sure you really do bend them at obtuse angles, which is where they are at their weakest. This could potentially get him to release and back away, but it could also make him angry and come at you even more, so do be ready to get into the Fence and continue defending yourself once you've escaped.

So that is a little bit of the direct escapes to work free from his grab. Have a go at them. Begin gently and lightly over a couple of sessions until you've got the technique and then you can start going a bit harder with them. Just don't rip your clothes if your training partner is holding on too tight!

So what about indirect escapes when you don't target directly the technique that is being applied at you?

You might kick him in the groin. Poke him deep into an eye socket. Scratch his hands or face or eyes. You might Stiff Arm him, hen Palm Heel or punch or elbow him in the face and into his nose.

Basically do anything that you can to get him to release you. You can combine all these things, direct and indirect escapes.

And don't forget to keep shouting. Someone might hear you. Shout and shout again.

But the above techniques really are great. They're good enough for professional judo and jiu jitsu athletes, so they're good enough for you and me to know and practice so we can avoid grabs or escape them before we can get dragged somewhere.

BEAR HUGS FROM
THE FRONT AND THE REAR

If you are grabbed in the bear hug position you are really starting to move into the deeper fight areas now but we are going to consider it here as it is something that can happen early too.

The grab around your torso/waist is an indication of something more serious. In itself the bear hug doesn't hurt or cause you any damage. It is what it implies - that you're about to be taken away to another location or you are about to be toppled to the floor - that is where the fear and urgency comes from and this is what we have to stop from happening.

You might find yourself in the bear hug if you are ambushed, where the man just grabs you and that's the first you notice of him. You're in a bear hug right away, in other words, as soon as things start.

You could find yourself in a bear hug if a man approaches from the rear and you didn't manage to deal with him, which is covered in Part Four, in the chapter Man Approaching From Behind.

A bear hug could be used against you at any time once the conflict has gone physical and he wants to take control of you. He might suddenly grab you to stop you from hitting him or from escaping if you're trying to get away.

In the bear hug his arms are wrapped around you like this, either from the front of the rear.

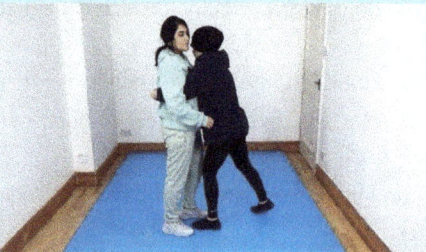

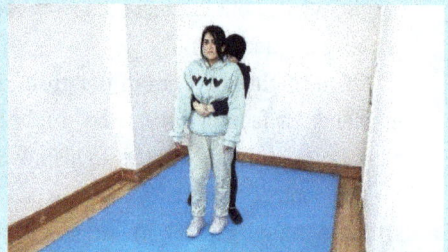

His arms are tied up in the action of the bear hug and so he is less able to hit you but your arms are free and able to move on this occasion. (We will cover the restricted arms position in a moment).

Let's escape the front bear hug. First you need to get this shape as shown below.

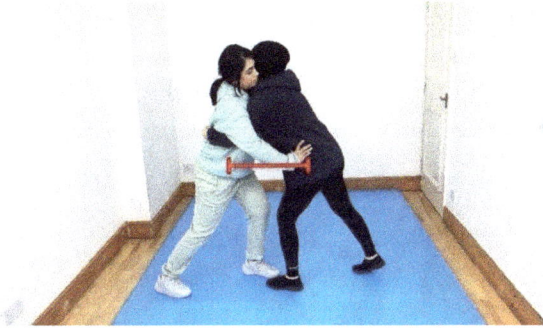

Note how you are pretty much in The Fence position but this time your hands are on the waist of the Bad Guy and not up protecting your face and neck.

So, you're roughly in the shape of the Wide Fence.

Feet square. Hips dropped down a bit. Your body structure is solid and strong. You're balancing well on your feet. And this time your hands are not up protecting your face and neck from being hit, but are being used to push at him.

He is trying to lift you up or move you about but to do that he has to get a tight grip. He will use this to control your body, squeezing you in towards him. So we need to prevent that.

There are several things you need to do - at about the same time.

The first is that you forcibly and strongly push your hips back and keep them there away from him and towards the ground. By doing this you keep him from controlling your hips. It is only when he takes control of your hips that he really has major control of you. Up until then he is mostly scrambling for control.

So create a decent gap between your hips and his (as shown by the red line above) and maintain that gap. If you lose that gap, fight for it and get it back. It's really important. He has to have your hips to really control you. He might be subconsciously aware of this fact but it's likely he doesn't actually know this.

You'd have to have served your time in wrestling to know such a thing.

So he won't be ready for you to just move your hips out and keep them there.

You can push on his hips to create the distance of the red line. You can push with both hands or just the one.

By getting your hips (your Centre of Mass actually - one of The Magic Five) away from him makes it far more difficult for him to lift your weight. By dropping your hips you also make it far more difficult for him to move you about, especially if you've got solid footwork to keep you there and prevent you from slipping and tripping.

For you to get a little better understanding of this, take a look below. Do you think it would be easier to pick you up if you were in Position A or Position B?

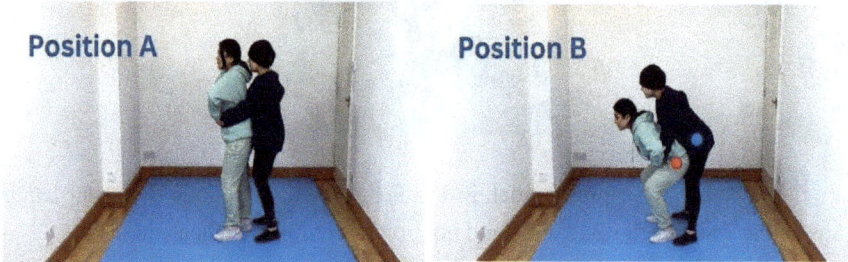

Obviously, it's position B which is more difficult, right. There are several reasons why, such as mechanical inefficiency etcetera, but the one concerning us right now is very simply that your centre of mass is much lower than the Bad Guy's. The red dot shows your centre of mass (which is at about where your hips/navel area is) and the blue dot shows Bad Guy's centre of mass.

So you automatically knew that B would be much harder to lift. So anytime someone wants to lift you up, quickly drop your centre of mass lower than theirs and you are now going to really cause them issues.

I'm digressing from bear hugs here, but actually even if someone is trying to throw you to the ground you can pretty much stop them by lowering your hips suddenly to the ground. It really is something worth remembering.

But let's return to bear hugs from the front.

You've dropped your hips, and are pushing on his hips to create separation. What you are also doing is putting a lot of pressure on his fingers and hands now so they can't grip as effectively. He can't lift you or drag you about if his grip is going to break any second. So he has to make sure he has that grip. First before he can do anything to you.

So this position really does stump the attacker very quickly.

And now you are in position to fight back and escape.

You could use a hand to attack his face or groin or whatever else you can do but note that it will be a scrap. He will be trying to get you to break your posture. You will be trying to maintain it or get back into it. This situation will not be neat and tidy in real life.

There is a chance that he might let go immediately, but there is also the chance this could be a struggle too and continue for a while.

So you just have to fight your way out. After that back away, keep your Fence and stay ready in case he comes back at you. Be VOCAL and keep moving away if you can.

So that was a bear hug from the front. What about from the rear?

The most important thing you need to remember is that the concept is the same as above.

You are going to try to achieve the same things, but the execution, the way that you get to them, is a little different because of the positioning.

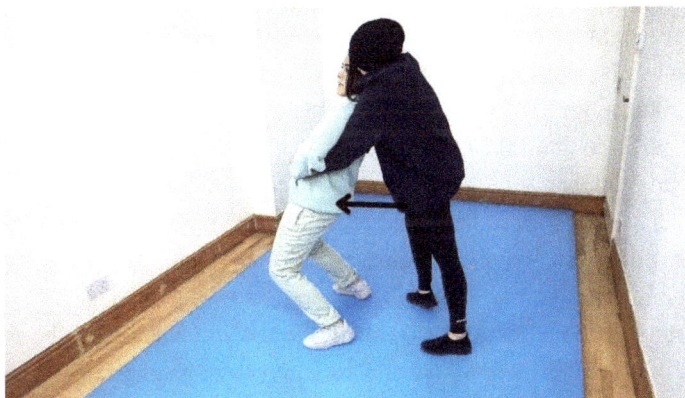

Again, you're trying to create a distance between your hips, as marked by the black arrow above. You've dropped your hips lower than his. But this time you can't push against his hips with your hands to keep him away - and this is where it is difficult to describe in a book - you push your upper back against him and at the same time you push your stomach forcibly against his hands so there is pressure there on his hands. (You must tense your stomach muscles as you do this otherwise it won't work).

Make sure you keep your balance so he can't take you down nor lift you up.

This time, due to where you are, you can actually push down onto his hands to apply further pressure onto his grip, like below, and this increases the chances of breaking away from him. I personally find the rear bear hug no more difficult to deal with than the one from the front. From the front I will go for his face and groin to distract him or to hurt him, and from the rear I will go for his hands and groin.

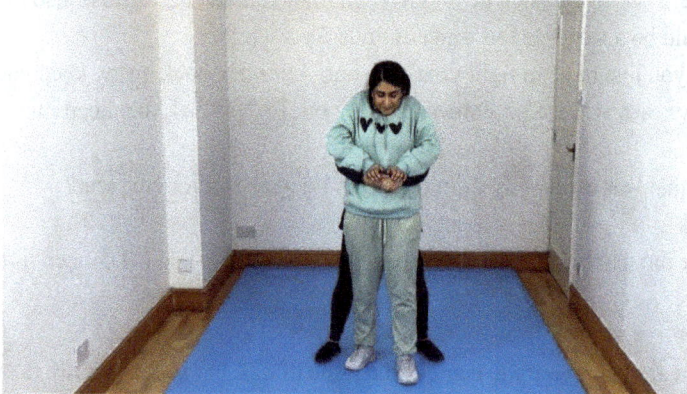

Drive down with both your hands. Aim to apply continuous and pressure with your hands and your stomach. You will be challenging his endurance to grip and it's difficult for him to lift or move you about until he's got proper grip. I've practised this move a lot and I usually manage to get my opponent to let go very quickly but to do that with a strong person you have to apply continuous pressure to the hands and then apply sudden, explosive pushes with your own hands too.

So you suddenly push hard, and repeat several time, never letting up on the pressure you were applying already anyway, and neither losing your stance/stability.

He might still not let go with that but I know you will already be scratching the back of his hands by now and making sure you're getting really deep enough that he's going to have to leg go.

When he lets go, push his arms down and away.

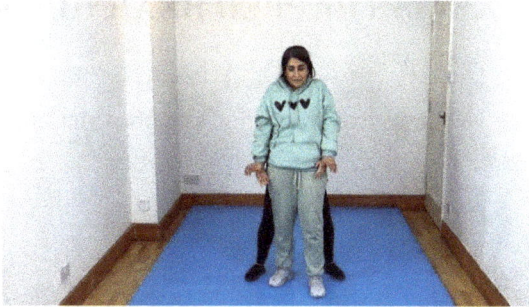

And now you will need to step away and turn round to face him immediately. Of course you'll be getting into the Fence and moving, whilst being ready to deal with anything he can come at you with.

A couple of extras before we move on.

Don't let him drag/drop/pull you to the floor and don't let him lift you up. You need to be ready AND to react to him doing either of those things. You need to react quickly and drop your weight if he tries to lift you up. And if he tries to drag you downwards, dump you to the ground, you need to keep your balance and push with your legs to stay up.

These escapes work as early escapes. If you're aware of him going to grab you, whether from in front or from behind, immediately fight him off by stopping his hands from gripping and jump into the escape position from there.

And if you're facing him, even if he's pulled you in, you can potentially play with his face. Give it a little tickle or something more severe. It's up to you.

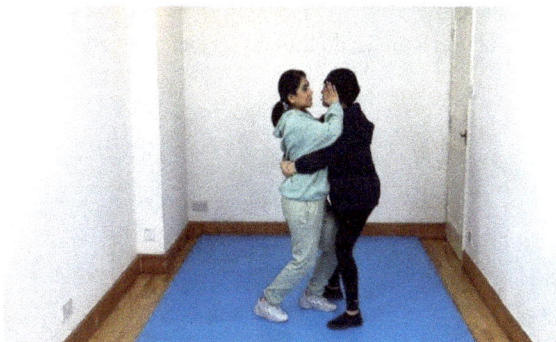

ARMS TRAPPED BEAR HUGS

So that was all with your arms free. What if he's grabbed you and your arms are trapped like this below?

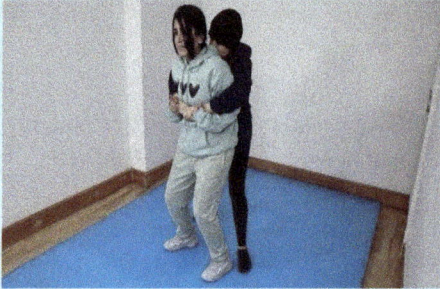

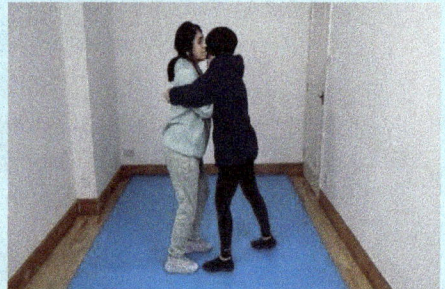

It's the same principles mostly. Drop your weight/hips so you can't be lifted easily plus move hips away to create distance and apply pressure on his hands by pushing against his hips if you can or by grabbing his hands as shown and pulling them down continuously like you did before. You might have the opportunity to reach down to his groin where you might be able to hit or pinch or grab and twist, much of which will depend on what he's wearing. But he might react as you move towards that area anyway and that could give you a chance. You could also reach up his shirt and do some deep scratching across his stomach or chest or nipples or neck or back. And you may have the opportunity to bite as well, especially the chest or shoulder/neck/face if you are facing him.

But you first need to quickly find the safe position whereby making it difficult for him to lift you or move you.

So from the front you want to do this if you can.

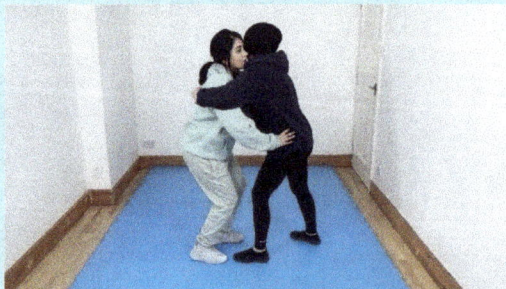

And from the rear you do this.

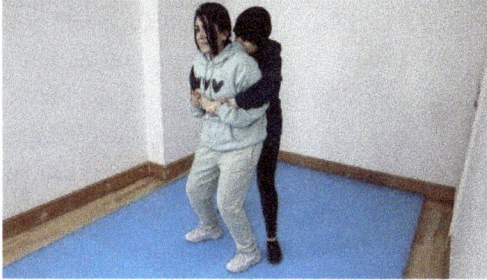

Note how Rahilla is getting to the Bad Guy's hands here. In this case grabbing and pulling them down. Engage your big lat muscles to do the pulling and not just your hands and arms. You'll be far more powerful that way.

Again, obviously you have indirect attacks too, so reach over to his face and whatever else you can get to.

QUICK TIP TO REMOVE FINGERS

Something you've probably thought about is having a go at his fingers.

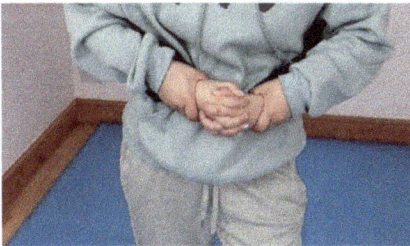

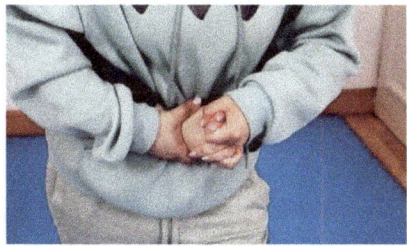

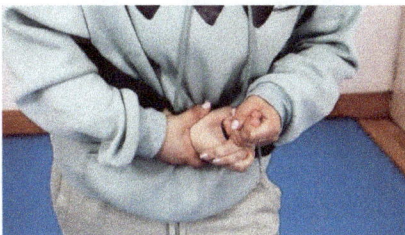

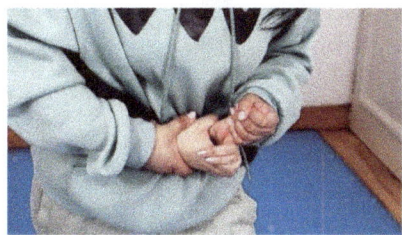

Whether it's one finger or two you're trying to deal with, make sure you have a good grip of it/them as shown. Use your whole hand against his finger/s and you've got a good chance of beating them.

Snap back quickly once you've grabbed them. A gradual pull to get them freed and under your control, then SNAP! It is best to also work at the angles that the fingers are not designed to move in. You don't just pull back, you arch the fingers if you can so they create a backwards C-shape, going against the direction they're designed to move in. Fingers don't like being pressured sideways either so bend them sideways at the joints. Aim to create a C-shape again. And you don't have to work on a whole finger either, you can apply the same techniques to any of the individual knuckles that make up each finger if that's all you can grab or the finger is slipping out of your grasp.

Once he lets go, move away, get The Fence and keep him at bay using strikes or the Stiff Arm or any number of ways that will deter him as you continue to get away from him.

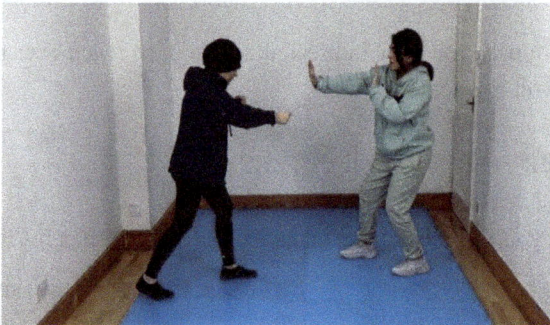

Shout, scream and be vocal as you move to a safer location.

HE'S CARRYING YOU AWAY?

"I've not had enough of bear hugs," I hear you say. "Tell me more."

"And what about if he's lifted me up and trying to carry me away?! What if I didn't get the chance to do all that stuff and he lifted me up before I could react?"

This scenario could arise if you were ambushed or any time he's grabbed you in a bear hug and you didn't manage to get things done in time or you didn't manage to do them correctly. It could happen to anyone; you or me. That's why we have to prepare for worse case scenarios even though our aim is to always get out even before a technique can be initiated.

The escapes for this are kind of similar to those above. The principles are the same with you taking on his grip etc. but you might start with the more visceral attacks this time - attack his groin, his face, eyes, ram a thumb deep up his nose, kick his shins, and just generally be uncontrollable.

You are now in a more dangerous situation. You are a step behind. He is carrying you to a new location and that implies real danger. So you do need to get visceral and very active right away.

You still need to apply continuous pressure to his hands so they loosen up, and/or you can go for his fingers.

You can apply the pressure in a few different ways too. You might push or pull on them directly like you would if you were still on the ground but you can also combine this with shaking/vibrating your body like crazy (shake/kick your legs and arms and body about). You can shake up and down too. It just makes it far more difficult for him to hold you up. It pressures his grip and moves his centre of balance about so he loses his footing.

Another thing you can do is you can lift up your weight by pushing on him and then drop it suddenly. To do that you first expand your body and become stiff like a heavy steel rod as you push on him and then suddenly release and become soft and unmanageable like jelly or cooked spaghetti. This sounds strange but it plays with his grip and moves your weight about so you're not so easy to move. You know how when you're holding a toddler who doesn't want to be held? That's exactly what they do. They turn stiff and you can't hold on to them then they turn into slippery (cooked) spaghetti and just slip out of your hands. That's pretty much what you're trying to do here but you're more advanced than a toddler and are capable of pushing upwards first if that possibility exists.

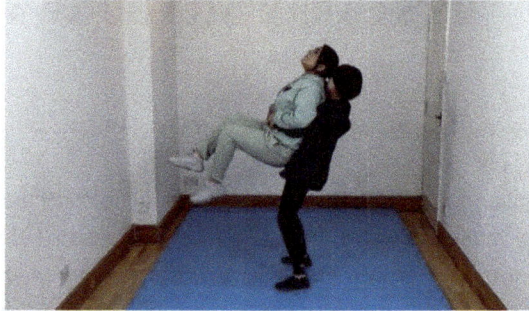

Shake away, become stiff like a board, repeatedly.

When you get to the ground be ready with your feet to get balance and base, and drop your hips low as soon as you're there so he can't lift you again. Continue fighting your way out.

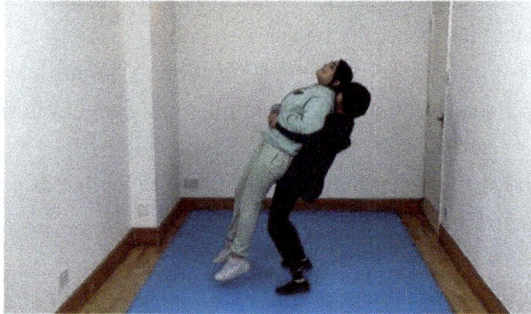

You again can reach for places to attack, such as the eyes, throat, groin and the back of the hands to start with.

EXTRA NOTES ON BEAR HUGS

With regards bear hugs you now have some highly effective techniques and strategy to deal with them.

But you have to be prepared and you have to have practiced recently to give yourself a fairer chance of dealing with them.

There are many more escapes too that you can find on TikTok or YouTube or even taught by martial artists. Some of these are quite fancy and look great in James Bond action movies. Most of them involve tripping up the Bad Guy and taking him to the floor, where on TikTok they'll show you some amazing leg-breaker you can apparently do, as if you were made in the mould of a Marvel

Superhero.

I don't know about you but in the really real world I don't want to be on the floor fighting with a guy if I don't have to be.

You know what? I know many of those moves too just like all of the martial artists who will be shaking their heads right now, telling me these trips and throws are available and how they'd fight Bad Guy on the floor and there are so many techniques to victory and I can beat my chest afterwards as I roar into the moonlit night of the concrete jungle.

But those who do self defence will tell you exactly what I'm telling you. That you may end up on the floor by accident but you don't want to go there really. If you find yourself there, you want to be fighting and escaping soon, getting up and getting away.

The fact is that in martial arts classes you have the liberty to try things out, and if it doesn't work then that's fine. You can try again next week.

For the competitive martial artist, at worst the referee will stop the fight if things get too serious. But in the real world? Choosing to take a fight to the ground on the chance that you *might* win? It's just silliness. I've trained a long time in the ground fighting arts, from wrestling to jiu jitsu, and I love training in them, but I really don't advise taking people to the floor by choice. It's a last resort at best.

So don't go there. You're starting to get some great skills to stay on your feet now, and should you find yourself on the floor, you're going to soon learn a move that gets you up very quickly.

Just in case you're still convinced by the over-impressive marketing by some of the Gracie Jiu Jitsu brigade currently taking place across the world, that you should take a man to the floor and do armbars and triangles and flying guillotines on him, I want to ask you where does a man generally take a women when he's grabbed her? Where does he want to go, especially in serious sexual assault cases?

The man wants you on the floor (or a substitute 'floor' like a bed or sofa etc). By helping him get to the floor are you not assisting in exactly what he wants to do?

It really does seem silly to me, and I genuinely can't believe that ground-fighting is currently being promoted as a self defence system in itself. You need to learn it and add a small but relevant portion of it to your toolbox but it is not self defence as a whole. Like with all the other big hypes throughout our lifetimes, this hype will also end one day. In the past it used to be Karate that was the only self defence, and then it was kickboxing. Everyone who could kick was doing 'self defence'. More recently it's been Krav Magaga but right now it's Gracie Jiu Jitsu. The flavour of the decade. This too shall pass - but I don't want you to get caught up in the hype along the way.

The only thing that is self defence is, erm, self defence!

So always aim to stay on your feet. If you fall, bounce right back up in any way that you can, or fight your way up. Get up, get away and stay alive. Go home and have a nice bubble bath with scented candles and a glass of your favourite tipple. Isn't that what you'd rather do? Or would you prefer to be rolling about all over a concrete pavement?

HE'S GRABBED YOUR HAIR

Other than limbs, clothes or bear hugs he could be grabbing you at the throat or he could be grabbing your hair.

Hair grabs are dangerous. They can occur at any stage and at any time in an altercation. They are an indication that the attacker has seriously mean intentions. At the very least he has massive control over you at the time he holds your hair.

You will not be standing up straight like often shown in social media click-bait videos on 'self defence'. But you know that. You will be in immense pain, bent over, off balance and being dragged or moved about like a rag doll.

This is how hair grab escapes are usually shown.

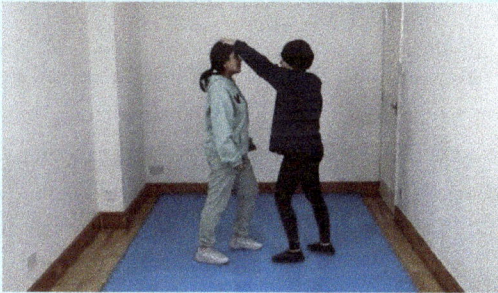

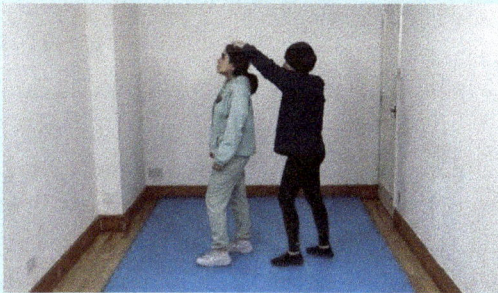

It's all very nice and tidy. Like you're heading out for a picnic and Bad Guy is just making sure the rain doesn't mess up your hair.

But this below is more like what a hair grab looks like, even though these are obviously staged photos.

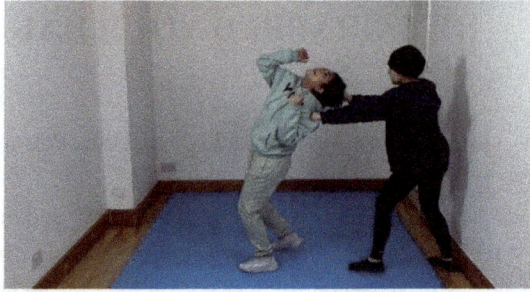

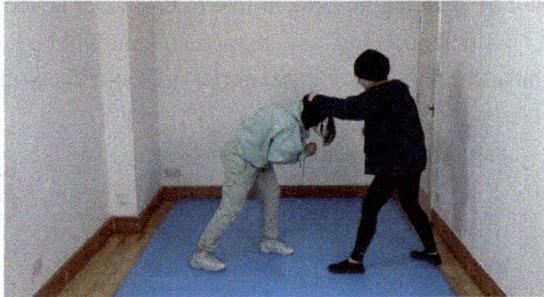

Hair grabs can be difficult to escape. You won't be standing still for long because he will be applying pressure and so you will be moving about. You won't be in a good structure/shape to defend yourself, especially at the start, when being pulled or dragged by the hair and you could easily fall to the ground or to your knees.

A hair pull is also super painful. The pain might take over your body and mind. I know because back in the days when I used to have hair, it was pulled during altercations a few times.

There is something visceral about a hair pull that you have to understand. It is mean and it has intention. Intention to hurt you, dominate you and take you somewhere. A hair pull is combined with something else - being hit, strangled, or having clothes removed with attempts to sexually assault. A hair pull, in other words, can be damn serious and darn dangerous.

To give yourself a chance to escape a hair grab you need to deploy a full set of tools from your toolbox. You have to be able to get balance (using The Fence), you have to be able to hit the person with pretty much all the shots you can think of, depending on where you are and where he is, and you have to go to direct and indirect attacks interchangeably and quickly.

Without having a lot of ability and a lot of knowledge, the hair grab is really not so easy to get out of.

Luckily though, you've already learned some of the skills you need. Once you get through the rest of this book you'll be even better equipped at dealing with hair grabs (and everything else for that matter).

Right now though let's cover hair grabs.

First you need to understand that Bad Guy can grab your hair with one hand or with both. The next thing to understand is that this will either be close to your scalp or further away. Once he has grabbed the hair he then has to pull it to take control.

So all those things have to be in place for the hair grab to work.

Again we have the avoidance and very early escape possibilities. If you are aware that a hair grab is going to take place you can act early to avoid it. Knock his hand away (using a cupped hand, like shown in the grabs escapes). If he actually manages to get hold then you still have the chance to do this if he hasn't fully secured the hold yet.

So to start with just cup your hand and whack his hand, wrist or arm away and prevent him from grabbing your hair. You obviously add indirect defences to this, hitting him, moving out of distance and suchlike.

Should he have secured your hair with a good grip then there are certain things you will need to do.

If you are still on your feet then you need to firstly deal with him actually pulling your hair and taking you off balance. Once this is in place, once you have a little balance and control, you can start working on fighting him off. But without these in place, you will get dragged around and struggle a lot more to deal with him.

If he's grabbed near your scalp you need to move your hands so they rest on his and then clamp his hand to your head.

Something like this.

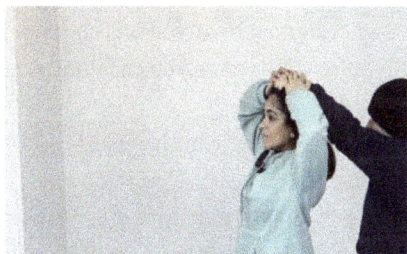

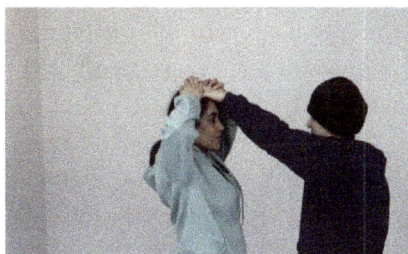

This is for demonstration. In reality you might be bent over and very uncomfortable. He might be holding you with two hands in which case you might be able to cover only one of his and deal with that first before moving to the other.

With your hands on top of his like this, pinning his hand down tight, you're now in a position where he can't pull at your hair so easily, though you might still be in pain since he still has hold of you hair. He could still pull you and you could fall over or be dragged and that's why you should also have moved into the Wide Fence to get some balance and stability too.

He might be pulling you about at this time but by keeping a low and wide Fence and by clamping down on his hand you can actually start the fight back.

If for some reason you can't actually get to his hand then take a hold of his arm and keep it secured so he can't use it to pull your hair.

So once you have a relatively stable position you can go to his fingers and hands to attack them or you can go for indirect attacks too. (When I say a stable position this does not mean static. You are still in the fight and there will a tonne of things going on).

To go for his hands and fingers you can scratch the back of his hands really deep, or you can grab a finger and twist it at an obtuse angle. Think of how a finger works. Now bend it in all the directions it doesn't normally work in. There are quite a few ways you can bend that finger. If one direction isn't effective, switch to anther.

You might also be doing indirect attacks at this time. The Groin Kick is a decent possibility here, so are Palm Heels and attacks to the eyes, for starters. Talking of starters, you might get a chance to bite his arm or something else too. Keep fighting until he lets go, then back away, get your Fence and stay ready to deal with anything else that comes your way.

So that's if he's grabbed you at the scalp. If he's grabbed your hair further away from the scalp then the process is the same again but the application is slightly different.

Again you need to have some control of the hair pulling and you need to have some control of being dragged away (or dragged to the floor) before you can fight back. You don't need full control but you do need enough so you are not being dragged away and being kept off balance. If you're off-balance you can hardly do anything effective at all.

So first control the hair pull. You can do that by grabbing his hand or wrist or even the arm that he is pulling with and hold it in place so he can't pull (too much). You don't have to grab by the way. You can trap it too. Push it up against him or pull it against yourself and hug it tight and now you are taking back some control of that hair pull. Just get control of it any way you can.

Next, or at the same time, get The Fence and get your balance, and now you can fight back right away in any way that you can.

My advice is to get visceral. The hair pull is a nasty thing and it's no time for civility. Go animal from the off.

If you have keys or a pen then maybe this is the time to unlock his face or draw a moustache and funny eyebrows on it.

Jokes aside, this is a dangerous and serious place to be. No joke.

Something to note is that when the hair is actually grabbed it will be entwined between his fingers and it's all going to be very difficult to untangle. It's very difficult to just pull his hand off. You have to attack the hand and fingers or attack some other part of him to make him loosen up and let go.

So you can see now why I teach hair pulls really late into my lessons. You really do need to know a lot of the basics before you can really get out of it.

But just go animal. It's up to you. But the hair grab is a very serious situation in my opinion.

Just a final note, when girls fight girls, the hair grab tends to be quite an Early Fight situation. The situation will go from a verbal altercation straight into a hair grab. Or it will be a punch followed by a hair grab. I know you don't hang around those kinds of people or places where this could happen to you but I've seen it happen randomly on the streets a few times because one female glanced accidentally at the other, who read the glance as some kind of dead-stare challenge. I've seen this even happen in daylight. On all these occasions the girls did not know each prior to their chance meeting. So do be ready if a girl approaches and an aggressive conversation starts. Your hair is probably the first or second thing she will aim for. So block her before she even starts. Get out of reach even before that!

In short, if someone has managed to grab your hair, stop them from pulling it, get your balance and go animal. All of this right away. That's it.

Make sure you build your foundational skills too as that will ensure you can escape earlier and more easily.

SCRATCH LIKE A SCAREDY CAT
(AND COLLECT DNA)

Scratching isn't just for itches or kittens. We all know how to scratch an itch but let's add a few things that make it a more effective weapon.

In situations that don't require too much force, let's say some fella is annoying you but it's not a 'serious' situation in that it's not violent, it's just pressured enough that you need to make him move. You can scratch as normal, not too hard. Maybe a 'normal' scratch will do, send the message, and you can leave.

But scratching can also be used more effectively in times of real need. You might want to scratch his hands to make him release them when he's got a proper hold on you. You might scratch his face or anywhere you can get to on the body, the body, the torso, the legs.

Where there is skin there is a scratch.

Here's something you may not have thought about - scratching is one of the best ways to collect evidence against him. Scratching leaves skin particles under the fingernails and these will have DNA which can be used as evidence or used to catch him afterwards if he is not caught immediately.

So a nice deep scratch is good, to collect DNA.

In a serious situation, to make the scratch most effective, you really do need to scratch like a fighting cat. Deep. Repeating. With purpose.

So get your nails in deep. Use the strength of your fingers to do that. Curl them up and dig in. You need to have a strong hand. Hold it like it's made of steel.

Don't just use your fingers to do the scratch either. Get those big muscles of the arms and lats, and get your bodyweight behind it too. A powerful swiping action done like a tigress would do it. That's what you're looking for. The tigress might appear to use only her arms (or are they legs?) but she's not. Her whole body is involved. Watch next time you see a house cat going for a scratch. The whole body is employed behind the action.

So you need to be a wild cat.

Note how a cat in a fight doesn't stop at one scratch either. It attacks continuously, rabidly and repetitively until it is safe.

You can use one hand or both; alternating one and then the other; or both together. You can hold/press his face or limb in place (to a wall or floor or held in any way that you can) with one hand while you scratch good with the other.

Scratching isn't likely to stop a fight though. It's likely to cause a reaction you can use to break away or do something else with.

It also shows you're ready to fight back and it disrupts and delays what he is trying to do. So do scratch if it's appropriate to do so.

You were going to do it anyway. I just wanted to remind you how good it is.

If you create a solid structure with your hand, something like this picture, hold it like it's made of steel, and then use your whole body to scratch - you will get a more useful scratch.

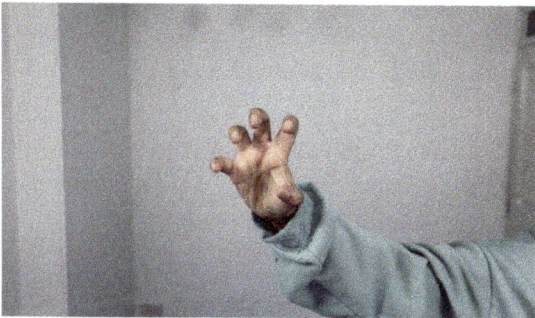

To save yourself, scratch down his eyes, his face, into his nose, his stomach, his hands, his scalp, or anywhere else that presents itself.

Get real deep and repeat and repeat again until you are free.

Be like a big bad scaredy cat.

BITE LIKE A RABID DOG

CAUTION

This chapter is quite excessively violent and contains gory details so please be advised. You can always leave it out completely or come back another time. This is your book so do what suits you best. It's just I had to include this here because I think it's quite important information. But you have been advised that it is somewhat gory.

Scratching isn't just for itches like biting isn't just for bananas.

The same applies to biting as does to scratching in some ways. You can give warning bites if the situation is less serious. But if it requires it, and you can control your squeamish, you can bite very deep.

I'm sorry to put such an image in your head. But you don't need to think about it right now. We are talking about any time you are in serious danger, you can do what you have to do at the time.

There are different levels of biting.

Bite and Release. A bite often gets a reaction. This is because we intrinsically know that a bite can have serious consequences if done severely. So just trying to go for a bite could buy you a second in which you can do something else to help you escape. In less serious situations you can make your intentions known by biting and releasing Even if you bite it isn't likely to stop a determined attacker but it could make him think twice about continuing to attack you.

Here's the thing though, once you bite someone, they won't give you that chance again. You might get lucky but it's more likely they won't let you bite again. Not the same area anyway. It's such a powerful move that they will do anything to avoid it.

So your one chance to bite needs to be successful and do what it needs to do at the time.

Why are you biting?

Do you want to just deter him or get him off you?

Do you want to hurt him so he knows he's in for a fight? Or do you want to maim him, so he can't continue?

What you want to achieve, will determine how you bite.

You can bite very early in a confrontation, if you get the chance. Or you might bite towards the end, when things are dire and you think you might lose your life.

I've already said you may get only one chance to bite. The thing to remember with a bite is that it's one of a few things that could actually end a fight, depending on the level of damage you have caused with it. In other words a bite could genuinely save your life if done correctly so you need to make sure you know how to bite.

This is not a nice lesson. We're about to go animal. Hold back your squeamish for a second or maybe skip this for now if you've heard enough of biting and come back to it another day.

I remember the first time I discovered the biting martial art, called Kino Mutai, and the shock I felt at what they did. When I first watched the dvd I actually put it away and said I'd never do any of that. It was just too much. Biting like that went against my civilised mindset. It just took things to a whole new level and I actually didn't watch the full training dvd until I went back to it about a year later. Over time I became somewhat desensitised to it though the dvd is not on my regular viewing schedule.

So I don't want you to be shocked by this but I also want to give you great advice that you can use, so continue at your own risk! You might decided to watch it and do what I did - which was put it away but kept a note of it in the back of my head that this was something possible in the worst of circumstances.

I don't like this much! However, I'm sure some of you will be salivating and this will not cause you any problems at all!

So let's get the gruesome bit over with.

When you're biting, for the reason of saving your life, you need to be biting chunks off and spitting them out. And you need to be biting again and again. And keep spitting. You need to go savage. You need to bite through muscles, tendons, veins and even small bones. Right the way through, and keep going until you know you are safe.

You need to go rabid.

That's the only real way you're going to get the person off. This level of vicious action is very likely to stop him entirely, depending on where or what you have bitten. Depending on how deep you have gotten or how much area you have covered or bitten off.

Note that we have an advantage over most animals too, in that we can hold the area we are going to bite. If you're going to bite his face or neck you can hold his head, secure it and bite away. If it's his arm you can do the same. Secure it first, by grabbing it and keeping it close to your mouth, or secured by pushing it onto him so he can't move it, or against an object/the floor or a wall. Secure then bite and you can keep biting for longer as he can't just move the target out of the way.

I'm sure I don't really need to give you the targets to get at. Basically anything that is protruding and is close to you is a good target. Most often the nose, ears, lips, jaw, cheeks, tongue, neck, trapezius muscle are available at the top end of the body. The hands are also usually exposed so you have the fingers or the sides of the hands and even the wrists potentially. His arms might be exposed, from the forearm, up the bicep and all the way to the shoulder.

Other parts may be available but will often depend on the clothes he's wearing.

There is no significant seasonal variation in any type of attack on women. Attacks occur through the year and the weather doesn't reduce them, so he could be wearing a thick coat in winter or a thin shirt in summer. The coat will prevent any bites to the chest but the t-shirt won't.

So bite what he gives you. Whatever is closest and you can get access to is usually what you should start with. Secure it and bite away. Otherwise trick him and grab access to something. Pin it and bite as much as you can.

And brush your teeth afterwards.

Just to make sure you understood the method, I'll tell you that in the practice of Kino Mutai, they actually get an animal carcass and hang it up. They then grab hold and literally, rabidly, bite (and spit out) chunks of it like a wild animal. They will not just bite one small area but literally cover as much as they can. This is what they did for when they were standing up.

For training on the ground they attached steaks (using string) around their partner and then they bit that to shreds! I'm not suggesting you do this, and I'm not saying they are crazy because I know they do this for reasons of creating reality etcetera but I want you to just understand that there is a whole lot more to biting and that should you have to use it then you can use this knowledge.

Push away your civility for a bit and live if that's what it takes for you to go see another sunny day on a beach in Greece.

As a side note, if you're feeling sick then just go for it, preferably all over him if you can. It's been documented many times that vomit is one of the things that puts men off from attacking a woman - though it doesn't seem to be the case in serious sexual assaults, where it appears the man can still continue even with vomit on him. But if you've bitten bits off him then hopefully he won't be too keen to also deal with vomit and you can get away.

Not a nice chapter, was it, this one? I do apologise. But hopefully now that you have this knowledge you have actually been made a little bit safer.

THE STIFF ARM TECHNIQUE

The Stiff Arm technique is something else you might do automatically, just as you might scratch or bite, and I'm here to hopefully help you develop it into a more successful technique.

The Stiff Arm is just that - sticking your arm out, making it solid, so that someone is held at bay and prevented from getting closer to you, prevented from doing things to you.

It is one of the single most disruptive things that you can do - which is why you would probably do it automatically anyway.

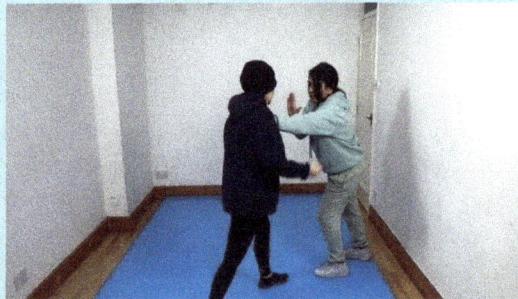

Here it is just pushing Bad Guy away with one hand to keep him at bay. This would likely be a quick push and then you'd move back into The Fence if he backs off. If he doesn't back off then you apply the Stiff Arm again and hit him with the other hand a few times, preferably Palm Heels to the face and forehead.

The Stiff Arm just seems so mundane. So unimportant that you wouldn't pay any attention to it. It's not sexy like a punch to the jaw or a snap-kick to the groin. But you would be under-estimating its value. It is like a car tyre. It doesn't do much, does it? Just a bit of rubber that goes round and round. Boring. There are many other things in the car, like the panoramic sunroof or even the sunglasses holder, that are more fun than the tyres.

But depending what tyres you have will determine so much of your driving experience, far more than any panoramic sunroof ever will. The tyres are what will get you out of snow or stop you aquaplaning when you're doing 72 on the motorway in the rain. They determine noise levels inside the car and stopping distances in an emergency. If a tyre bursts it could send the car flying into a ditch because you drove over a beer bottle and hadn't checked the condition of your yres before you set off on the journey.

But tyres are just boring. The Stiff Arm technique is the same. But it is actually a proper self defence and martial arts technique that can be used in so many ways you're unlikely to have considered consciously. You can use it to Get Up as shown here if the person is between your legs (but check the chapter on Get Up). You would sit up, push against his chest or face and then Get Up.

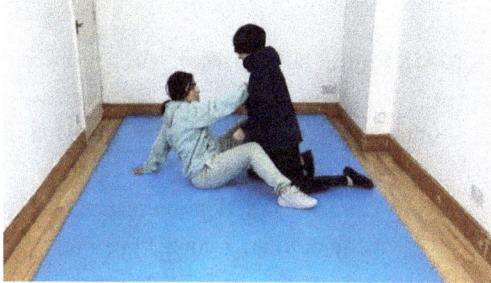

You can use it in most other ground positions too. You could use it as an early move if you end up on the floor.

As he comes in to secure a hold on you, you stick a Stiff Arm out to keep him at bay, and you Get Up or Shrimp out etcetera, as shown below.

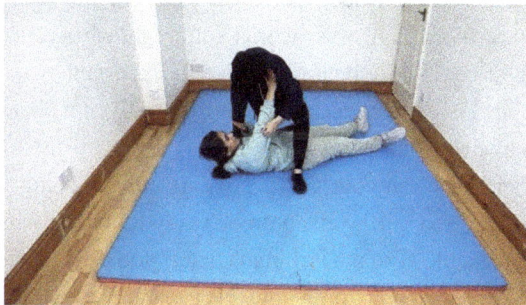

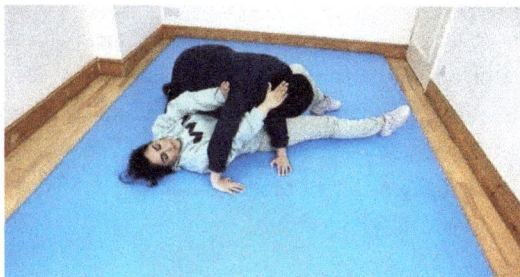

So you can stop him getting on top of you and start your escapes.

The Stiff Arm is just one of those things you will use all the time.

It is often a transient technique that you use to get to other things. You use it to push him away so you can escape. You use it to hold him at a distance so you can hit him. You can use it standing up or when you're on the floor, whether you're underneath him or on top.

Remember you used it to push his hips away when you were bear grabbed?!

It is actually an absolutely essential technique and one you should have in your armoury to deploy right away.

Along with The Fence, Palm Heels and grab escapes, it will help keep you on your feet and make it very difficult to drag you away or take you to the floor.

In judo the players absolutely hate the Stiff Arm because it neutralises most judo throws. You just take hold of their jacket at the chest or shoulder and every time they move towards you to throw you, you Stiff Arm them. They really don't like it, although it is a legal move and fully allowed in judo.

Here are some details so you can make it more effective.

When the arm is straightened, the elbow might or might not be locked out when you do the Stiff Arm. In other words you might have your arm completely straight or it might be slightly bent. But what is important is that you hold this position very solid. That's what makes it a stiff arm. Even with a bend it needs to be held like it's made of steel.

But remember that when your arm is sticking out and being solid that he can whack it at the elbow and hurt you, so do be ready to instantly move it or stop it being solid and breakable. The other thing is that if you stick your arm out at him, he will grab it, but you already know how to escape that, or you could Palm Heel him repeatedly if that's a better option.

It's one of those techniques that's very difficult to explain in writing and so easy to show live or on video. It's a technique that is very easy to undervalue. After all, all you're doing is sticking your arm out and making it solid, aren't you? Yes, that's exactly what you're doing. But because you can do it in so many different places, at so many different times, and thwart so many different attacks you cannot underestimate its applications.

Just sticking your arm out at him (at his body or face or anywhere) will often make him change tactics and delay him.

One of my favourite ways to use it is in attacks. Whilst standing, you push on his face with your hand, and as he twists to escape that, you get a good knee to his groin. He was too busy concerned about his face for a millisecond and you used that to your advantage.

Or you push on his face with a Stiff Arm and he can't see your other arm piling a Palm Heel right into his jaw.

So start practising it now in The Fence to begin with and later you can add it to the ground positions when you get there.

With your training partner, or even on your own, get yourself standing in The Fence position and move about. As your partner, who is playing Bad Guy, moves forwards, you suddenly stick your arm out and Stiff Arm the Bad Guy in the face or chest. If s/he backs away then that's fine, keep moving away. If s/he doesn't then hit them.

You can progress onwards and get your training partner to grab your arms when you Stiff Arm and then you escape from that and then hit them.

Have some fun with it, add some of the other techniques and play around. That's how you'll make it yours.

THE GET UP!

Anytime you hit the floor you should GET UP. I think I've said this enough times now.

Use whatever means you can. Scramble. Fight. Drive your way up. Anything you can. Get to your feet. Do not stay on the ground if you don't have to.

Beyond just doing whatever you can there are a few technical ways of getting up and they're all worth knowing in the long term but the Get Up is by far the single most important of them all.

If you hit the floor any time - you can use the Get Up to, erm, get up.

So here you are on the floor, flat on your back. Bad Guy is standing up.

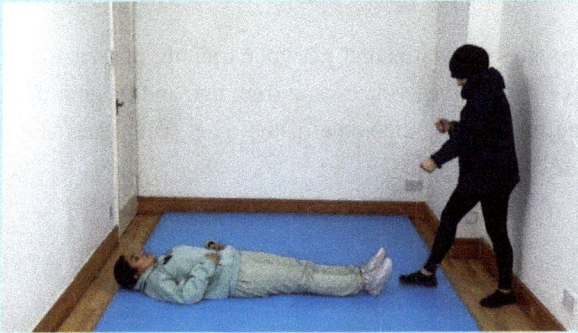

You should never realistically be in this position for long, if at all, but for training purposes we are going to start here flat on your back.

The first thing you do is put your arm up to protect yourself. So you put that arm somewhere between your head and Bad Guy, as shown by the yellow line. Whilst you do this, sit up, planting your other arm down to the floor, as shown by the green circle.

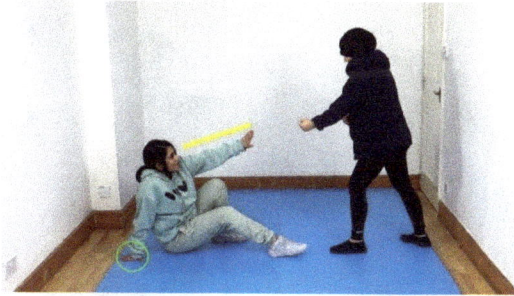

Note that you also plant down the foot of your opposite leg. So in the picture above, the arm planted is Rahilla's right arm, and the foot/leg planted on the ground is the left foot, so it is opposite arm and foot.

Now you need to push off with your planted arm and foot so that you can move your other leg (right leg back and plant it close to your hand, as shown by the purple arrow). So it's something like this.

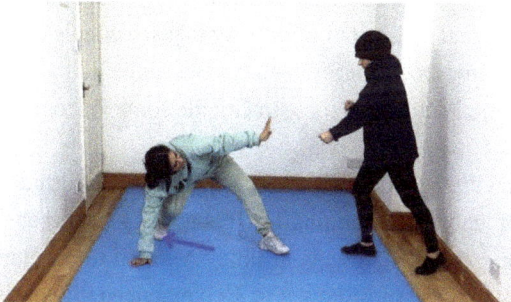

And from here you can stand upright, and move away as you get into The Fence.

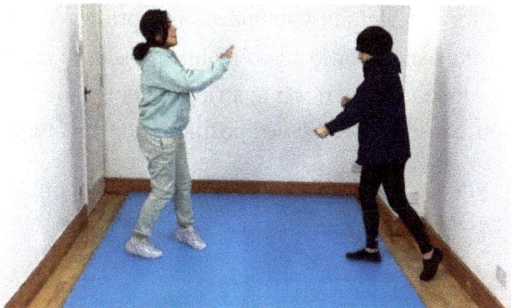

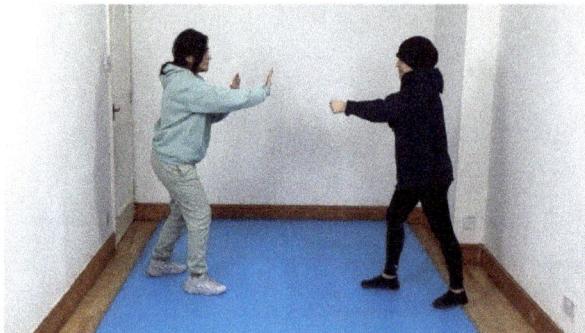

And that is the basic version of the Technical Get Up (which is also called The Stand Up or Technical Stand Up in the martial arts).

There are several variations of the Get Up. Some slower and with more moves for those who are less flexible and less able at the time (which will happen to all of us at some time, won't it?) and versions for those who are more athletic, which include jumping back and getting out of the way in just a couple of moves. They're not easy to describe in a book, unfortunately. But above is the standard version that is used all the time. You're welcome to Google some videos on it and see how to do it there.

The Get Up, as with most fighting situations, is often performed with stumbles and trips and lots of unbalanced getting up. It is not as graceful as we'd all like it to be. So whilst you practice it, take your time. Allow it to develop. Allow flops and fails and stumbles. That's just how it is. I've practiced it a lot (like with most things that I do) and I still end up tripping over my own feet sometimes when I do it under pressure, if the opponent charges at me or something. So to start with, just practice the move without pressure. Then slowly get your training partner to make it a bit more difficult for you and put you under some pressure. This is the single best move to get you from the floor to standing up and is used thousands of times every day across the globe in martial arts sparring sessions. It's that good.

It is a move you can use from other positions too but requires skill and

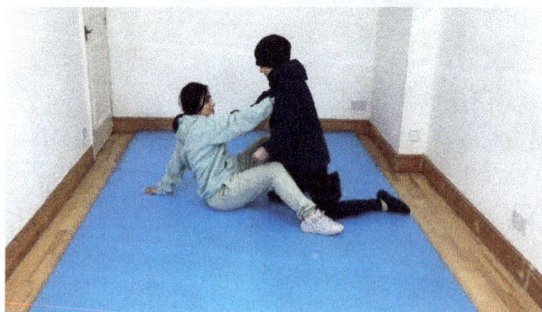

practice. For example if someone is between your legs, you can Stiff Arm them as you sit up and then you're already in the Get Up position, like in this picture.

As with most the techniques in this book, do what you have to do. If you're on the floor and you need to get up, then do what it takes at the time to do that. It is your mindset, your attitude, that will make your brain come up with the things you need to achieve the goal you set.

It may be that you use the Get Up along with other techniques. You might hit him first with kicks or Palm Heels. You might bite him, and this is what gives you the opportunity to Get Up back to your feet.

It might be that you scrambled up and in no way did it look anything like a Get Up. That's all fine too. It's just that knowing it properly means you've got a more superior chance to adapt it and escape. So practice it. Learn it really well and turn it into a skill you own. It's a good cardio workout too. Try doing 30+ in a row and you'll see what I mean!! Go on! Try it!

STAGE FOUR: THE DEEP FIGHT

This is now the deepest territory. The good thing about it is that very few know how to fight in this area proficiently. Every man, and probably even monkeys, can punch, but fighting on the ground requires skill and thought to be good at it. Even in the extremely unlikely situation that he has some skill on the ground these techniques in this book are the exact ones that are employed day after day across the globe to beat skilled fighters. Skilled professional and non-professional fighters who know these techniques are going to be used against them struggle to keep these from working. I'm talking top of the fighting food chain. These are the top skills in the world as used by world champions and legends of fighting.

Here's the thing though, to beat those guys at the top you have to train for years, take the right amount of protein (and a lot of enhancing substances) and did I say you need to train for years? Yes, I did. But still these are the same techniques that work against those guys - though usually by someone who is as strong and as trained as they are. You and I are not going to be able to beat them, but we don't want to. They're not the people we need to beat. That's not our game. It's rare for a martial artist to go around being violent. Think about all the people training martial arts and in combat competitions every single day across the globe and you occasionally get a story of one who's attacked someone. It's really rare.

The people who attack you (and me) tend to not have a clue. Rather than physical fighting skills they are usually living by guile, deception, experience and attitude (their drive/resilience). And so I have found them easy to beat once an altercation actually goes physical. Like, I have literally been surprised at how easy it was sometimes to deal with people. I was used to fighters. I spent time with them every week since I was a kid. So when it came to dealing with people on the street in my police career I was shocked at how easy it was to trip them or hold them down etcetera and I got myself a reputation amongst my police peers as someone who could handle himself. I mean, I can - that's what I trained for and got bruises and black eyes every week learning. But where I'd spent most of my spare time since I was a teenager, everyone had that reputation and each person could harm you if you weren't on your toes. Very few were singled out in the dojo like I was now in my police career.

That doesn't mean that I wasn't scared during those times or now if something happens on the street. I find myself covered in sweat and shaking afterwards. And yet each time I virtually didn't exert myself at all and if any real danger arose I would have put a stop to it quicker than their mamma's would have liked.

Yet here I am, a veteran of having put literally hundreds of people under my control when I needed to, never failing once, and I'll still be sweating and shaking after an event today.

So the point is that these skills really work BUT you must practice them and remember that you will be scared, especially scared if you get into the Deep.

Knowing the skills is a great start. Knowing them and having a bit of a go at them (practising them) will begin to give you an idea of how things might feel should things ever head downwards. But practice - and I mean recent practice - will keep you out of much trouble. And should trouble start, it will get you out of it much quicker than if you hadn't practised.

Here in this section we will cover the skills you need in the Deep Fight. We won't cover specific situations, because these skills apply everywhere, so we'll stick to the street scenario as it covers everything we need. But do have a think about how you'd use these skills in any places you visit that concern you. Maybe it's club you attend or you go to the beach on your own all the time or maybe you drive for a living and have to have people in your car. These skills can all be adapted to those situations.

So here you will deal with the Deep Fight. The one where you're now stuck - for a short time at least if not for longer. But a place where you will know what to do and the Bad Guy won't be expecting it.

THE FIGHT FOR YOUR LIFE;
TO THE DEATH

So at this Stage you didn't manage to get away from him, for whatever reason. It happens. It could happen to me as much as it could happen to you.

It could be that you've gone through all the Stages - early avoidance failed, then he spoke to you, then he grabbed, then you had a scuffle standing up, then you went to the ground and so on.

Or it could be that you were ambushed and the first you knew was when you were thrown to the ground or grabbed in a choke from the rear. It can happen.

It could be you were asleep on a towel in the park or lying in a hotel room and this is the first you know of it, and you're in deep already. I'm not trying to scare you, but just to show that there are a lot of ways that things can happen, so just know this and you'll be less shocked by it. I don't want you to be too surprised. I want you to kick ass and take names.

So this is the Deep Fight and you are a little stuck. To escape now requires a few more moves than at the earlier stages, which is why this is called the deep fight. You might be on the floor or you could be trapped when standing too in the Deep Fight. It might be he got behind you and is choking you. Or it could be you're on the floor. The point is that with the earlier Stages there were less moves needed and it was a little less scary. You were less trapped. You could have broken away a lot easier. Now it's going to require more effort to get out and it's probably going to be much more scary.

So, we're going to deal with it and make it a little less scary.

I'd like you to remember that, although you are apparently more stuck now, you still might actually get out of it as quickly as you came into it. That's a nice thought, isn't it?

Let's aim for that, but also deal with the fact we might be trapped for a little while too.

Here's another good thought to remember - that the Bad Guy won't be staying here long if you get here. If you can hold him off, he will most likely bolt soon. He doesn't want to stay. It's very rare. So hold him off and most likely than not, he will be gone and you can get to safety. All the skills you learn here will help you do that but these are also the skills that help for the longer situation too.

GROUND FIGHTING POSITIONS

Before we start, we have a tiny problem to talk about when it comes to teaching ground fighting. Even to teach the essential moves on the ground requires several books because the area is so vast, so I'm only going to cover the basics here. It also takes a good couple of months to learn all the necessary escapes and get the essentials on the ground.

But I'm not going to leave you totally unprepared and unprotected here. Far from it. You're going to get a lot of knowledge, it's just that it can't all be fitted into one book. If there is demand for this then I'm happy to write a book just covering that area and I currently do teach this online and in person but it's over a longer period of time. It requires time commitment to want to genuinely know this and it demands a bit of work from those who want to really learn it. That's another reason why so few people know how to fight properly on the ground, because it takes time and commitment, and so it was quite easy for me to deal with them out there on the streets and homes of London.

What we are going to do here is going to take you so much further into that arena and I know if you practice this next set of skills, that you'll be able to deal with most situations. It might be those few extreme situations where you might need more skills, that's all. With practice, you'll be able to deal with most scenarios.

So let's get on with building some amazing skills in the area that probably scares you the most…

The ground.

When you are not standing, you are considered to be in the arena of 'ground-fighting'. This is a specialist arena that was something no one was interested in 30 years ago. Everyone wanted to punch and kick and a few wanted to throw people. Very few wanted to mess about on the floor. I happened to start training in it when it was just getting noticed, about 25 years ago. At the time there was a variety of ground-fighting martial arts, from Catch Wrestling and Shootfighting and so on, but there was a family from Brazil who pushed things to a new level. The Gracie family had discovered Judo and were bringing it to the 'West' but under a new format. Instead of fighting standing up, which is what most of what judo is (throwing) they took the ground-fighting components of judo and blasted them ten levels better. They called this new system Gracie Jiu Jitsu. I was lucky enough (along with my brother Saeed) to be training judo at the Budokwai judo club in London at the time when Gracie Jiu Jitsu first came to the UK. It was coached by this early 20's shy guy called Roger Gracie. He coached at the club along with his father, Mauricio Motta Gomes, although the official coach was someone else they had put in place. So I started learning jiu jitsu at an early stage when I was still in my 20's. What I didn't know was that Roger would go on to become considered the greatest jiu jitsu competitor of all time. I can see why too. I was okay at fighting. At the time I had been training for a while and was decent at much of what I did. I could handle my own against most, even competition level fighters. Roger came along, we grappled, and I felt like I was fighting a tonne of steel. He could run me over anytime he chose. It was really interesting to spar with someone that no one seemed to able to handle.

Literally no one. Upstairs at the Budokwai were world and Olympic level judo players and he twisted them up like rag dolls. Later came a time where literally no one in the world could handle him, except maybe his uncle Rickson but that match never happened.

Roger is a very likeable man but I've always preferred his uncle Rickson as a fighter and coach. Rickson Gracie is a philosopher and a cerebral fighting machine. Many say he's the greatest fighter of all time, including the greatest street fighter of all time. He would enter backyard fight competitions doing what was called 'the Gracie Challenge' and it is reputed that he never lost. I have followed Rickson and his methods from the start because he was more into self defence and wasn't really a competition fighter. Within the ever- growing Gracie clan, he's considered the one no one could ever beat, even in sparring. We are talking literally about the best of the best.

The reason I tell you all this is that I have been doing this for a long while and by sheer coincidence I started with the person who is considered the greatest ground competitor of all time, so I learned quite a lot back in the day, even though I didn't quite realise how exemplary it was. I also trained at London Shootfighters, where the coaches were again pretty much at the top of their wrestling game, and I've been a part of the great Dave O'Donnell's Elite Fighting Systems, where they did plenty of sparring on the ground, which included strikes as well as submissions.

So I've learned a lot but what I did learn though, I realised later, was way more than I really needed. I've said this many times already. It took me years to master ground-fighting but in reality I only really needed to master about five to ten percent of it. If you can get good at this small amount of the really good skills here on the floor you really can become super good in this area and you will have very little to worry about.

That's what I'm trying to say.

Rickson Gracie says that only 20% of all jiu jitsu (which is a pure ground-fighting art, as I have stated) applies to self defence. The rest is for competitions or for show. I think it's even less than that which you would ever need to use in reality. I know this because I have real world experience of it unlike the tens of thousands of people who teach jiu jitsu and other forms of ground fighting every day across the world.

So I want you to be confident that you can handle yourself on the ground. Because you can. And you don't need to know all fifteen thousand of the jiu jitsu techniques as sometimes advertised.

I know I am emphasising this a great deal. But this is the place most women fear being the most. Because it feels like a very vulnerable place, where you're dominated and overhwhelmed and you don't know what to do, like an upturned turtle on an ice skating rink.

But it's actually not like that once you become familiar with it. In fact, you'll find the attacker is actually the one who is unfamiliar with it then and doesn't have a clue. And again, I say this from decades of expereince actually dealing with violent criminals. Most of them - almost ALL of them - have no skill on the ground and just blag and power their way through it. So it's a place you really can become familiar with and it's worth it because it's also where the man eventually wants you when it comes to sexual assault or other violent assaults.

But, although I don't want you to be scared, I want you to remain apprehensive of the ground and try not to go there. But should you end up there then be 'comfortable' and know what to do.

So welcome to the ground and let'!s get comfortable with it!

THE MAIN GROUND POSITIONS

We'll start with the main positions you could find yourself in. These all appear quite scary to be in but we'll deal with that as we go along.

You've hit the floor. The good news is there are only a limited number of positions you can find yourself in and you're about to learn them here.

When you hit the floor you might be on your back, on your front, or on your knees. That's it. There is no other way for you to be on the ground.

So let's start off with the most dangerous and most scary positions - the ones on your back. I call these the underneath positions of ground-fighting because in all of them you are underneath , with him on top in the more dominant position.

This below position is called the Full Mount. The Bad Guy is sitting on top of you, either upright or leaning forwards.

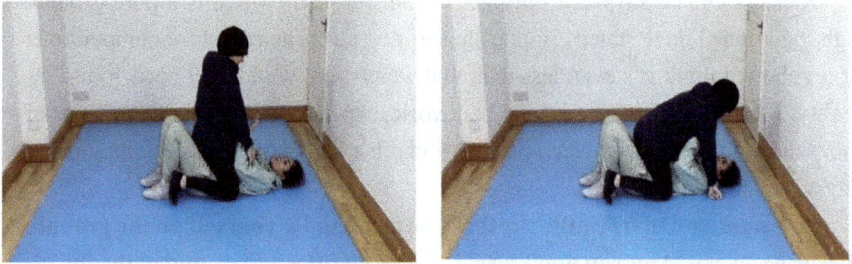

This is a very scary and claustrophobic place to be.

I want you to have a go with your partner (or just imagine it on your own. Spending time on the ground gets you more familiar with it anyway). Get your partner to sit upright on top. Get them to lean back. Get them to lean forwards. Whilst they do all that, you should feel where their weight is. It is to the side? Is it leaning backwards? Forwards? Have they put weight on you or is it on their knees? They might not have put much weight on you!

All these considerations will allow you to feel where he is weakest and strongest. Where you can push him off or where you can slide away from him. You are actually starting to work on the principle of Sensitivity, which is one of The Magic Five actually. You will understand this better if this is your second read of the book. Right now just get a feel of what the person on top is doing. Get them to move around and feel where they are weak and strong.

Then swap over and get on top yourself. Have a feel of where your weight is this. Think about where you are quite weak here or where you are vulnerable. You're starting to now get a feel of these positions and your brain will automatically start to think of ways out without you even having learned any specific techniques yet!

Thank you, brain!

This next position (below) is called the Cross-Side. Here Bad Guy is at your side making a cross with your bodies. Either he is lying on top with his legs out or he is kneeling and a bit more upright, So again he can be upright with more weight on his knees or he can be leaning forwards with more weight on top of you

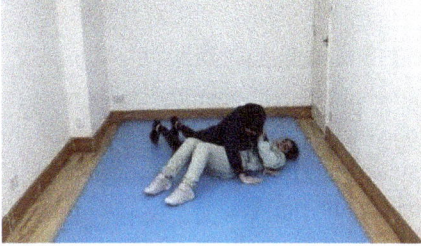

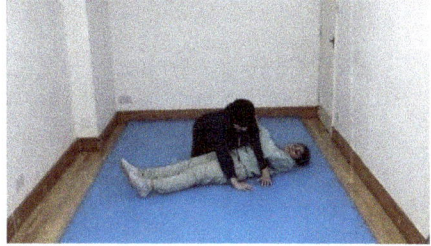

I'd like you to have a practice at this too. Feel where his weight is. Feel where he is holding you down.

Even more importantly, feel and think about where you can escape, where you might be able to sneak out because your partner is not pinning you down in that area and so there is less pressure that you can slip out from underneath. Where can you just push him off? Get a good feel and think about it. Get your partner to adjust positions a little. You'll notice that at any time he switches positions he is more vulnerable to you hitting him or pushing him off etcetera, because his mind is engaged on what he's doing rather than what you're doing.

Give him a bit of a push here and there and see how he reacts. You need to feel all this now and you can do these things in all these ground-fighting positions.

Let's move to the North-South position (below). Again he might be leaning on you with legs back, or be more upright or be on his knees.

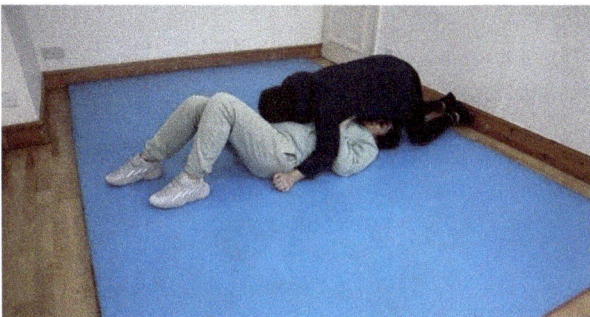

Again, have a go at the top position and the underneath. Feel where his weight is. Think about where you could escape, where you could push him off. Even think about where you could bite or do other things too! But we're going to go through all that in a while anyway.

This is next position is called The Scarf (or *kesa gatame* in judo, if you're into that kind of thing). Basically he has his arm around your neck like a 'scarf'.

Remember the headlock throw we did in the chapter 'Don't Get Thrown'? This could be the end result of that so you could also do that with your partner. Start standing and then GENTLY move your way to the ground into this position, so you start to get an understanding of the situation. You might learn how to escape early from both! (HINT: pop your head back! Just pull it out if he's not holding very tightly.

So it could be your were taken to the ground like this or it could be when you were on the floor he's reached out and got an arm around you like this. Anything can happen.

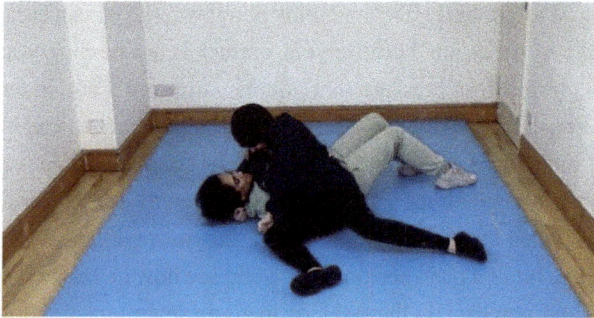

Please have a go at this too. Spend a five minutes underneath, and five on top. Feel his weight, see where you can slip out of, and even where you could palm heel or hit him in some way.

In this next position below he is between the legs. This is called The Full Guard position in the martial arts.

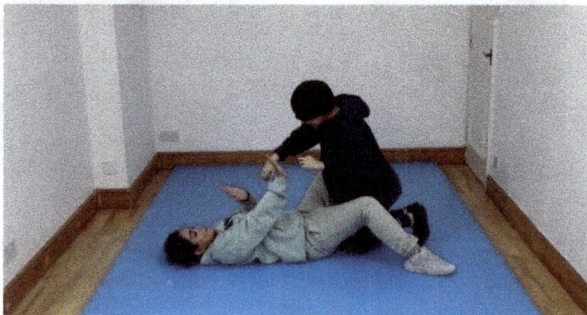

It is the favoured position of jiu jitsu fighters. They actually seek out this position to fight from it. As in they might be in a different position and they *choose* to get into this position. This is another reason why I don't agree with jiu jitsu being a complete and perfect self defence system although that is how it is currently being marketed. You cannot choose to be here as a woman. That's just silly, isn't it? However, because Gracie jiu jitsu does work from here a lot, it means they have actually developed plenty of dangerous moves from this position. It is just that I really can't agree with the tactic of bringing men between your legs when you don't have to. Especially as a woman.

A major rule in self defence is that you should escape from the first position you find yourself in. Don't stay there and play games. Get out. Should you however find yourself in the Full Guard Position then you must work your way out of it, and for that purpose Gracie jiu jitsu does have a lot of valuable techniques. I just wish they didn't consistently seek this position to fight from in the first place. It's just not a good idea for women's self defence.

Again, get yourself in this position and think about it. Remember that you have a very good chance of using the Stiff Arm and Get Up from here. What else is there? What else can you do to escape? Where are your legs? Where are your arms? Where is his head? Where is his bodyweight? Have a think. Get familiar with the position.

Can you Get Up from here? Kick him in the body or head and Get Up? With practice, you can.

Next is the Half-Guard. You have one leg trapped and one free.

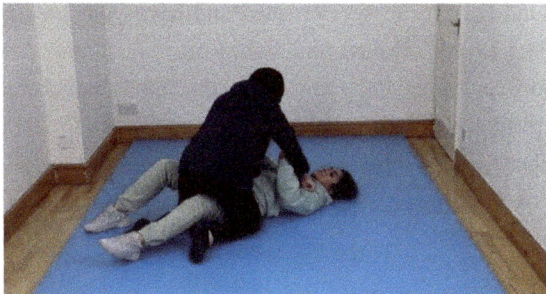

Have a go at this for a few minutes too. Settle in, get a feel of it. Now is the right time to orientate yourself here. Have a think about it. See where his weight is heaviest and where it isn't so heavy.. See if you can do a Get Up from here too. (You can, if you scramble, fight, slide your leg free and use the Stiff Arm but it might not be something you can do on your first few attempts in this position. But keep trying! Rome was not built in a day. It took about a week at least.)

So that's pretty much it with the underneath positions!

So, as you can see, there are not that many positions you can be in when on the floor. The thing to understand is that although these are the only positions you can be in, there are infinite variables of them. He might be upright or he might be low down. He might have a leg up or his legs down. He might be pushing a knee onto you. You might be on your side rather than on your back (which is a much better position to be. We're going to work on that in a second). He might have control of your arm or head or clothes. You might have his clothes or his head and be pulling them about. So there are infinite variables BUT they can only occur in these positions. These are the only positions you and him can be in if you're both on the floor.

But it is because of these variables that it can seem like there are a million things going on and it's all confusing when you're on your back with him on top fighting you. But the reality is that these are the only positions you can be in! And once you know how to escape from them, he won't be able to hold you there. He hasn't got the skills.

The other thing you already know about these positions is that they are claustrophobic. If he is resting his bodyweight on your ribs or diaphragm then you might struggle to breathe as well. If your lungs are being compressed you will struggle to fight. But now is the time to get a feel for those things and realise that although it is quite horrible, you're not quite dead yet, and actually it's quite the norm for ground-fighting to feel crushed and have your breathing affected. So now is the time to get crushed and figure out that it only takes a few small adjustments to free you up and you can breathe again. So get free and get a good feel of these positions right now, before they can happen to you in real life. Let's get one step ahead, shall we!

Next up, we're going to work on escaping these situations so we can stand up and get away.

ESCAPING FROM THE GROUND

Now you know the most common positions there are on the ground when you're underneath.

In fact, you also now know all the positions you might be on top too.

It could be you both went to the floor and you scrambled and you ended up sitting on top of him in the Full Mount. It may be you ended up at his side in some kind of Cross-Side position. So you have covered all the top positions as well as the underneath.

Your options from the top positions are to either stay there or get away and these choices will be determined by your current situation and the severity of that situation. Is it safe for you to get off and get away? Or are you in a locked-room type scenario and are forced to stay and fight? Is he holding you there and you can't get away?

So if you need to stay and do things then you have a lot of attacks available to you from the top. Pretty much all of what we've already covered, from Palm Heels to headbutts, elbows and more. You will need to maintain your balance whilst you attack from on top though otherwise you can easily be pushed off.

It might be right for you to get off him, because you'd be able to run away for example, and if you are able to then you could use those attacks as diversions. Alternatively you could use them to hurt him so he lets go and you can slide off. You could push his face or body away using a Stiff Arm and use that to get away from him when you're on top.

Maybe now, or soon, is the time to go over all this. Have a little practice. Get on top and find ways to safely get off, whilst continuing to face him. Keep your hands between you and him so you can fight off anything that comes your way. Do that a few times now if you can. You might be able to slide off or jump off him.

Next, get on top and now get your partner to mildly stop you getting off them. What are you going to do now? Try a few different things. If they're grabbing your wrists, you already know how to get them off. If they are holding onto your clothes, you already know how to get their hand off. You've been learning all these skills already and now you see how they have universal application too. You don't even have to learn many new skills! (That's how I designed this book by the way. It did not happen by accident!).

Once you have more confidence (and you've got some good mats on the floor) you can start to fight a bit more and get your partner to fight back. Now you'll start rolling about too and find yourself sometimes underneath and sometimes on top, but this is also another thing that can happen in the Deep Fight. You're on top then you're underneath. Then you're on top again and so on.

Please do have a go at all this. Even if you're on your own you can use a pillow or a foam roller and your imagination.

Let's go back to the underneath positions.

Should you find yourself there, the very first thing is that you should NOT be flat on your back if you can help it.

And you *can* help it. This position here is the one Rickson Gracie says you must always find and start your underneath ground fight from it. It is the strongest position to be in when on the ground.

This position also stops you from being smothered. It also reduces the amount of control the Bad Guy has on you and it gives you a chance to Get Up.

Any time you find yourself on the floor, you must to move your body into this shape as soon as you can.

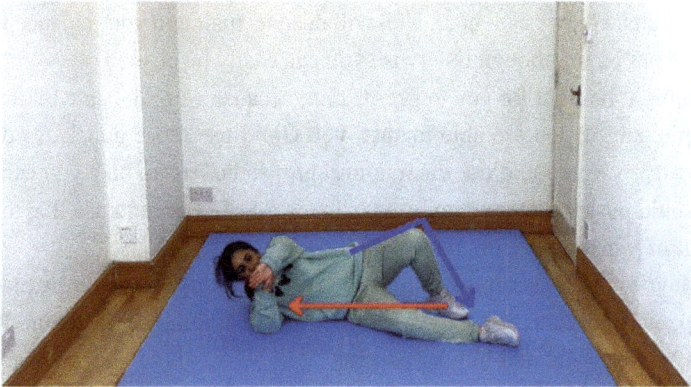

So do not lay flat!

It might happen though. It might be that as soon as you arrive to the floor you find yourself flattened. It might be that he presses down on you to flatten you, because it is easier to control you that way.

But do not stay flattened! Rickson Gracie says so and he knows what he's talking about more than you and me!

Move comfortably to your side.

Bend your leg and press your foot down (blue arrow).

Use this pressing foot to generate force all the way to your arms.

Your arms need to create a square frame like this that you can use to push off with and generate forces to hold off the Bad Guy.

This frame needs to be solid. It is without doubt the strongest position to be in, especially if the man is trying to put his weight onto you. This is also what you will need to do if you want to effectively push him away/back.

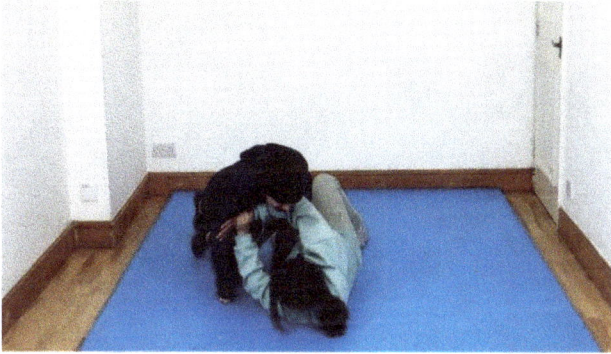

Here (above) for example, the Bad Guy is trying to put weight down but is being held back using this frame. Again, it is a position you will have to fight for but once you have it, you can do a lot more from it. For example you can move your hips away and start to Get Up.

A quick note about this position (which has no name that I'm aware of). Note that it is another transient position. You use it to block him for a moment and then you Get Up as he moves away for example. Or you use it to push him off when he is smothering you and then hold him at bay for a second while you do something else. So you might not be in it for too long. You might be in and out of it several times. Use it to get to other things or to stop him pressuring you for a moment or to let you breathe again. It might not be held for long but it really is a very strong position when you get it.

Have a go at it. Get your partner to press down onto your arms and push them away. Try it in other underneath position too. Use it to push him away so you can reach for his eyes or his face to hit. Have a play around.

There are times on the ground that you get stuck and you can't even fight your way to this position. In such a situation, where you might be smothered and overpowered, you need to generate power. Once you do that you can get to this position and continue from there.

"Yeah? How do I generate power in the first place?" I hear you ask.

Well, I'm glad you asked. To generate power you need to master The Bridge, of course!

The Bridge is what you use as the primary tool to create power on the ground. Not only does it help you generate forces, it can be combined with so many other moves that it is one of the most essential skills of ground fighting.
(In Brazilian jiu jitsu it's called The Upa. I prefer that name. Sounds more fun!)

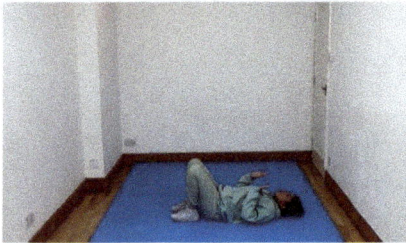

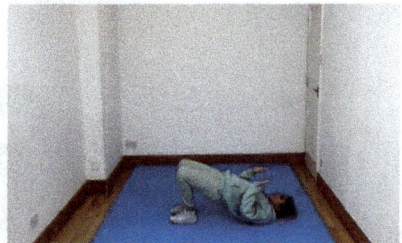

You start like this, with your leg/s bent towards your butt, and then you push through your feet and legs to drive your hips up high. You use the momentum you generate to push the person with your hips and also with your arms.
You can use it in most positions on the ground, for example if Bad Guy is sitting on top of you like this.

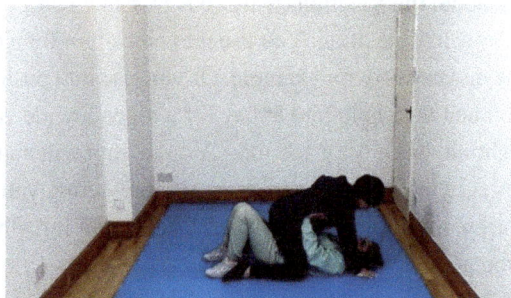

You bridge up high, whilst pushing at his torso

… …you push harder to one side…

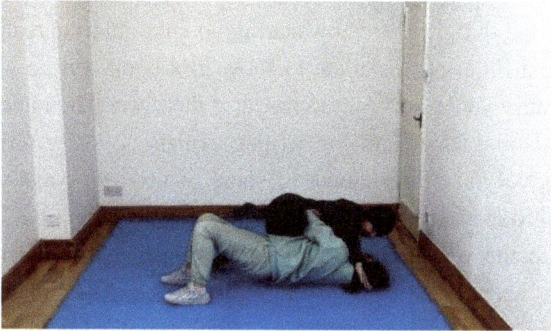

…and push the person off.

(You have to roll over to your front, Get Up and move away afterwards, of course)

But you can generate strong forces by using The Bridge.

Here it is from another angle.

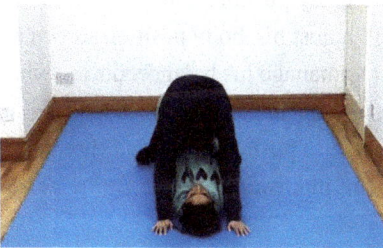

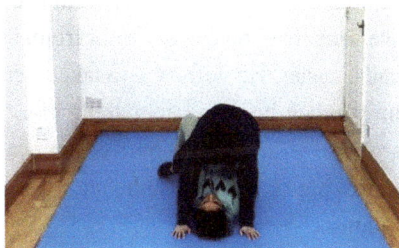

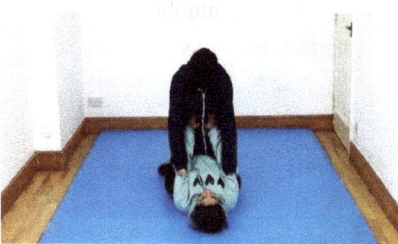

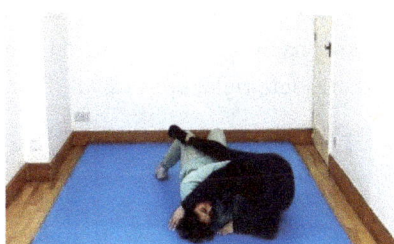

This above technique works and works really well. But against a man who weighs three times as much as you, are you going to just Upa him off? It's quite unlikely. You would need more skills to deal with him. You need to now start using the Shrimp move, Get to Belly, Get to Knees and combine them with all the other skills you have.

So here's the thing, we are now starting to enter into the realms of skills that are becoming a little too technical to show in a book. I'd be wasting my time writing it because you'd not want to read it if there were hundreds of photos and intricate details and accompanying writing explaining every tiny bit. So in this book I will give you a breakdown of some of the best ways you can use for escaping the ground but we are not going to cover everything. This book is an introduction to the whole concept of women's self defence rather than a full encyclopaedic textbook anyway. I might actually expand on it one day if the demand is there and people let me know. (But I'm not going to write a book if no one wants it. It's really hard work, you know!)

So we are going to continue learning some very important things that will carry you a long way in your journey of self defence but this is not everything that I would normally teach you. I'm working my way round skills that I otherwise wouldn't do.

So The Bridge, and its variations, are used in pretty much all ground-fighting arts, including American collegiate wrestling, Greco-Olympic wrestling, judo and many more. It is one of the most useful moves you can learn and apply.

Please make sure you have a go at it from every underneath position. Use it to push him off if you can or get him off balance. By pushing and bridging he will leave gaps that you can slide out from, he will adjust his body position so you can breathe easier. He will have to take a second to manage his balance, during which time you can be doing something else. And it may just be that because he's not ready, that you just push him off anyway. Use it to push him in every direction.

Talking of pushing someone off, here's an interesting fact about the ground positions:

Wherever Bad Guy is, he can only travel in a set number of directions. Whether he moves himself or you move him, he can only ever travel backwards, forwards, left, right, up or down. That is it.

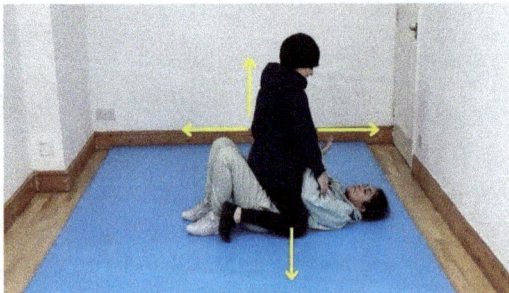

Here for example, on the Full Mount above, the arrows show all the ways he can go. So you can bridge and shove him into any of those directions.

The same applies in every position. Here for example when he's inside your Full Guard, the arrows show all the ways you can send him. With a kick or a palm or a push.

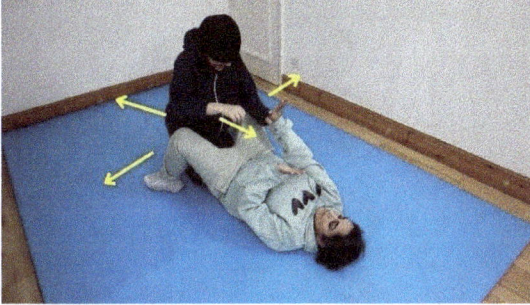

Guess what? These directions are all the ways YOU can go too!

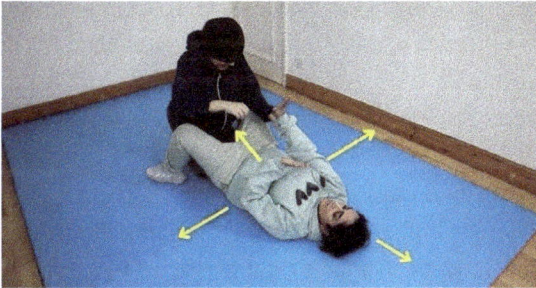

The arrows show all the directions you could potentially go to escape, or move away to if he's trying to hit you.

Scramble is the name of the game if you're on the floor.

Now, he might dominate you but he can't dominate you the whole time. There will be instances when he isn't in power - and we'll talk more about this in the chapter titled Moments of Power as we don't want to divert our learning right now.

Let's get back to showing you more arrows.

Should you manage to kick him away from inside your guard and he stands up, you can get into the seated position of the Get Up - and in this position you can actually move about. This will allow you some protection from him and allows you to scoot away to a safe enough distance that you can get to your feet.

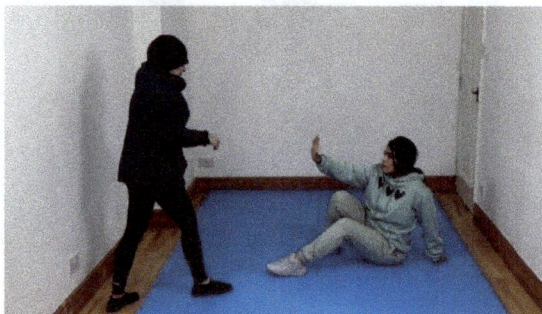

You can sit in the position shown and get your training partner to walk around you and you follow them, keeping this position and then Get Up as soon as you can.

Please have a practice at these things so they are ingrained in your memory. This will take a little bit of time and effort on your behalf but remember this is physical exercise and can also be a lot of fun if you have a well selected training partner.

You could actually do this on your own too. The Get Up is something I've done about ten thousand times on my own, imagining this exact scenario above, where Bad Guy is standing up and I've got to survive it.

Have a good go at it. It really is quite a super move. As a fitness exercise too as it uses up so many of your muscles, from the arms to the quads and the glutes, and it develops good hand-body coordination too.

So a final note with regards escaping ground positions. You need to wriggle and scrap and scramble. If he's on top, then bridge to generate forces to help you shove him about. If you can free yourself, start getting up and getting away. You can also hit when you're on the ground, and get visceral too. But that takes what?

You've guessed it - practice!! So have a play around. Enjoy your training. Do a million reps. Too much? Okay, a thousand will be fine. (Is it obvious I was once a gym instructor in this life?!)

Next up we're going to cover something we haven't mentioned so far, and that is 'the worst position on the ground'. Let's do that now.

THE WORST GROUND POSITION

There is one position that most consider to the be the worst on the floor, and that is flat on the floor, face down. If you are in this position and Bad Guy is not on top with his weight on you then just turn over and deal with what you have to. But if he's got on top then he can only be in one of three places and we have to deal with that.

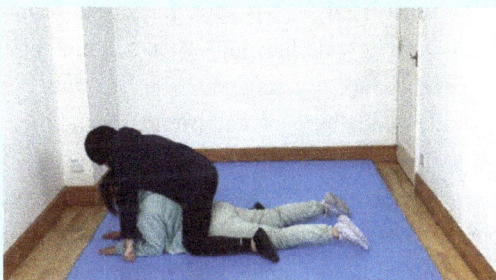

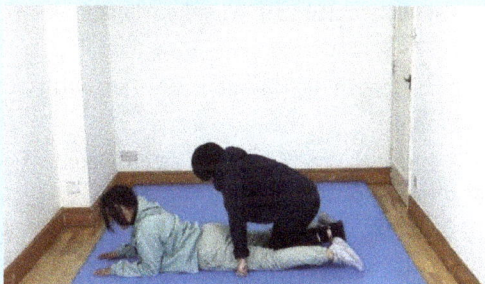

In this situation the Bad Guy could be between your legs, straddling one leg or sitting fully on top somewhere (either your back or your thighs/legs).

He might also be holding your arms down to control you. This seems to be a dangerous situation and to some degree it is but it is also not impossible to get out of if you know how. In training, I have found myself in this position hundreds of times and of those hundreds, I've probably struggled in it only a handful.

The fact is that most people who get on top of you like this usually feel they

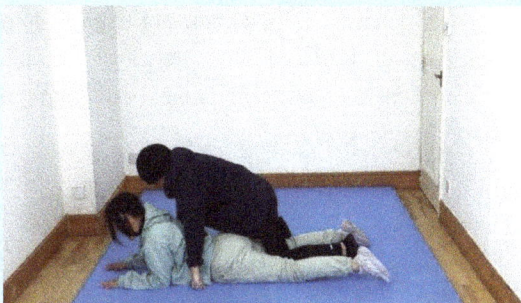

have total control of you and so they don't expect you to be able to get out of it, and that's much to our advantage.

But I am more equally sized to my foes than you might be to Bad Guy and I've got the tactics and knowhow of how to deal with this situation, you are saying, and you would be totally right.

However, the techniques and tactics that I use are just as applicable for you and I believe are good enough to deal with this situation.

The most important thing to note first is that you really need to turn and face him asap. No matter what it takes. It is safer for you to face him - and probably scarier - but you can definitely do far more when you are facing him. If you stay here then he has a good chance of doing whatever he wants.

So you will need to feel where his bodyweight is and then you need to travel the route of least resistance to turn.

When you turn you will be in one of the positions we've already covered and you can fight your way out from there. If you stay in this position you cannot hit him and you are purely being defensive and submissive. All you can do if you stay in this position, at best, is delaying what he wants to do. Your head and body are open to so many physical attacks. You are vulnerable to sexual assault. This really is not where you want to be. It is a bad position and you really need to turn out of it when you can.

(This position is one of the reasons why I say to people if you do judo to be aware of what you're doing. In competitive judo this is considered a safe position and so the judo player will *seek* it out on the ground because the referee stops the fight here and resets it. Judo is based on throwing the other person. Reaching this position in judo means neither of you can throw each other and so the game needs to be reset and you start again from standing. In the real world, seeking out this position as a woman (or even a man), might not be very sensible. It is situations like this where martial arts and self defence differ considerably sometimes. Imagine teaching someone to find this position as it's 'safe' from attack. That's what happens in judo).

There are a couple of other ways that you can use to get out of this position but they require too much explanation for a book so I'm going to direct you to our online course, which covers it in a couple more ways - but actually you already have the basic concept here, and that in itself will do you wonders in your process of escape.

Personally, if I'm ever in this position, I basically feel where his weight is. Depending on where it is, allows me to either move my arms or move my legs to try to escape.

Is he on my torso? Therefore his weight is higher than my hips, which means (since he is not putting his weight on my legs) my legs are free to move and I can potentially pull my knees towards my chest. So now I am kneeling and he is starting to topple forwards. If I can use my legs to power him off I have the chance to slip backwards through his legs and escape. I basically buck like a bucking bronco and try to shake him off, whilst at the same time I try to slide backwards so I can slip out between his legs. I find this technique works very well but it comes with the caveat that you really have to know Sensitivity from The Magic Five. You must feel where he is and what his bodyweight is doing all the time so you can shake it off.

If you've got someone really heavy on top then this is going to be difficult to do because they are just too heavy to buck off but just trying to do it keeps you in the fight and he might adjust his bodyweight and you can fight from there, maybe even turn to face him first.

What if his weight is on the legs then?

If his weight in on my legs then I tend to push off onto my elbows and then push my butt back to get to my knees. Now I am on my knees and elbows/hands and since his weight is either off me or only on my leg/s, I have some ability to turn or start to hit by swinging backwards at his head.

Both these escapes work well, when combined with feeling where his weight is, AND you need to make sure that you turn to face him and fight your way from there.

If he is holding your hands down and/or is sitting across your centre of mass, you need to become more technical and it requires a little more training but we are not going to do that here right now. Sorry! However, you know that you need to scrap. You know that you need to keep trying to turn towards him. You know that if he adjusts his weight you can bring your knees up and get to your knees. So you already do know quite a lot of how to escape, directly or indirectly, if he's on your back and is pushing your arms down. Let's move to a ground position we haven't covered yet though. Being on your knees.

FIGHTING FROM YOUR KNEES

So the first thing to note, that you might have picked up already anyway, is that all these positions are reversible. It could be you who is on top rather than him. The second thing is that many of the skills have learned already can be applied when you're on the ground. You can Stiff Arm and hit him so you can escape. You might need to bite or do any of the other attacks to get him off you or to set him up so you can do something else. You might need to break his grip on your clothes or limbs or hair before you do other things.

If you are on top and you have to stay until you stop him, then your options are to hit him with any of the methods mentioned before but now you really do need to know how to make him unconscious, which is a chapter coming up soon. You should know that if you are much lighter and much less strong compared to him, then you will struggle to stay on top unless you've practiced these positions. So you really could still be in danger if you're on top. At any moment he could throw you off so always be ready for that and ready to bounce up to your feet if you feel you're going to fall. It's better to be up than down.

So you need to know how to secure these top positions and then how to hit from them, and this is where the martial arts, such as judo or jiu jitsu will be reasonably useful for you. They don't do strikes of any kind but they do help you learn how to be in control from the top positions. If you do head that way, then learn how to hold these positions using good base and think how you can hit from there. You really don't need to learn the fancy moves like armbars and Ezekiel chokes and all that. They are moderately useful things at best, and require a lot of practice to pull off anyway.

Being on your knees is another situation you could find yourself in. This could be while you're scrambling to get up from underneath, or it could be if you slipped and managed to stop yourself from hitting the floor fully but ended up on your knees. It could be that he's dragged you to the floor but didn't manage to get you all the way there. It could be he's actually pushed you onto your knees. It could also be that you tried to Get Up and slipped and now you're on your knees. It could be other things too. Regardless of how you got there, you might find yourself on your knees when you are transitioning to or from the floor and so you should have a practice at this position to get an understanding of it.

Here are the positions you might find yourself on your knees.

You could be on what is called 'all fours', which means both your hands and knees are down. In this position, the person could be in front of you, at the side, behind or on top of you.

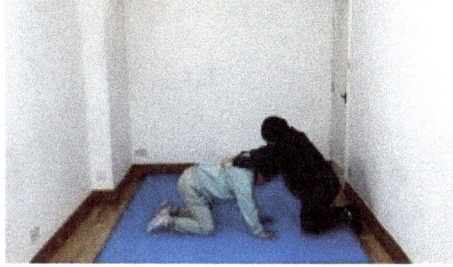

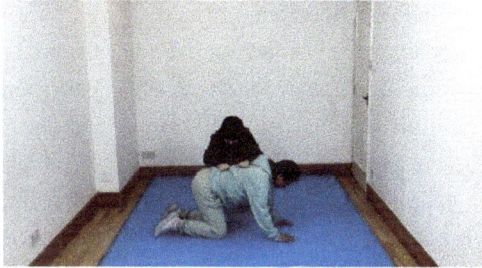

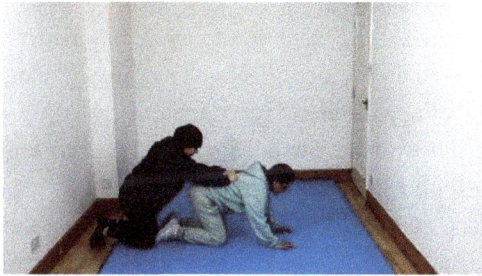

Another thing could be that you are on your knees but your hands are free. In this instance he might be standing up or he might also be on his knees as you both scramble.

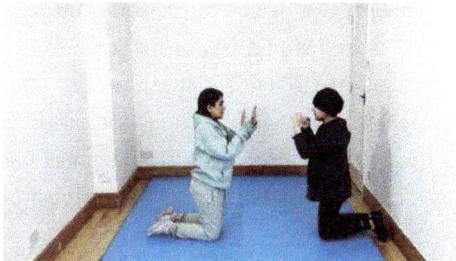

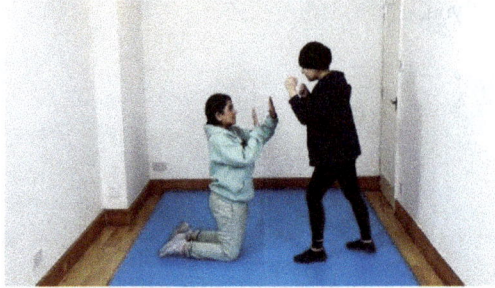

Or it could be that you are on your knees but he is stood up. Or vice versa. This might be because one of you slipped during the altercation, or it could be that you were both on the ground but one got up first.

So, all these positions are called 'on knees' or the modern jiu jitsu name for them is 'turtle position' if you wanted to search and learn more about them online.

In all these positions you can still only move in the same directions (back, forth, left, right, up, down). So you can actually move about. He can also do the same.

However, when you are on your knees you actually have far more ability to get to your feet. You are already on your knees. To get to your feet, just put a foot down, press hard and you're up!

Remember this. In fact I want you to try it. No matter where your training partner is, in any of the positions shown above, if you're on your knees, I want you to plant one foot down, push off and get up.

This will be more difficult to do if the person is on top and pressing down but actually it's still possible due to how strong the legs are. You might need to scrap your way out, and don't forget to face the Bad Guy and get your Fence up. You want your Fence hands up when you're kneeling anyway as it will be easier to react to anything he does, and also easier to hit him and do your attacks too.

This is worth practising because you will learn how to go from your knees to standing in literally a second. This is something you won't learn in jiu jitsu classes or anywhere that teach you to stay and fight and finish your opponent on the ground. But it is a fact that from your knees you are almost standing up and so you should because there are only two places you can go from your knees - up or down, and you know which of those I would favour for you.

You can sometimes put one foot down, then the other and stand up from there. Kind of squat your way up. If he's got his weight on you or has too much control that you can't rise with the power of just one leg, then get your second foot down too and then push up. And you can do it from all these positions, no matter where Bad Guy is.

Here's something else you might have figured out already: pretty much everything you can do on your feet you can do on your knees!

If you're on your knees, with your hands up. You can walk back and forth. You can hit. You can grab or push. You can (with practice) knee from here. You can even throw (grab both his legs like you would in a rugby tackle, keeping his legs together (especially at the knees) and topple him to the angle you feel he has least resistance). It all takes a little practice to be able to do it, but just knowing this now means you might try things in practice, which can transfer to reality.

I actually TKO'd someone in training from here, with a punch to the navel. I shot it right through him. Knocked the breath out of him and he couldn't do a thing for about a minute. In part it was because very few people know that you can do pretty much everything from your knees that you can from a standing position, and so he didn't expect me to punch anywhere except to his face. So he was covering that when I sent a powerful, driving punch into his navel and it had better effects than I had expected actually.

So get practising the knee positions and it will just be another place where you'll be more powerful than expected, giving you the advantage of being equal when he didn't expect it, but actually, probably, a couple of steps ahead of. That's where I like to be and I'd like you to be too.

HOW TO NOT GET STRANGLED

CAUTION

With regards practising, I don't want you to apply any strangles or chokes at all.

Because you don't know what you're doing you could seriously hurt your training partner or be hurt yourself.

WHAT WE HAVE BELOW IS FOR DEMONSTRATION PURPOSES ONLY. DO NOT COPY IT!

That is my official line for legal reasons.

However, were you to ignore my warning, to do this, where your training partner might put their arm around your shoulder/neck area, you should only work with someone you can explicitly trust and have discussed this with. I'm just trying to make sure everyone is safe. I know most of you are sensible so won't do this but for any youngsters reading this and who might be practising with a less mature friend (usually a male will be the less mature friend I'm talking about here) do be very careful. I don't want anyone getting hurt.

So if you insist on doing this, discuss with your partner, before you start, that there will be no actual strangling and choking and no squeezing and no serious attacks . You can actually learn a lot without strangling each other to potentially harmful levels.

I'm not going to teach you how to strangle here anyway, as I have said, as I just don't want to be responsible for injuries. I've had my throat hurt by zealous newbies several times. They didn't mean it. They were just too excited to learn strangling and ended up causing me pain for a few weeks. They went too quickly or just didn't have the awareness that I'd tapped and asked them to stop.

So my advice currently is for you not to practice the chokes and strangles, or only to do it with a trained and qualified coach only.

WHAT TO DO WITH
STRANGLES AND CHOKES

Well, this is not a nice place to be, being choked or strangled from behind, but again we actually have a lot of things we can do and, even more so, we have great potential to avoid this move altogether. It's actually not all that difficult, as you will learn in a moment.

The fact is that for years I haven't been strangled in training because these principles are very simple to action. In fact, just from this part of the book, and with a little bit of (very safe) practice you would actually become a hundred times more difficult to strangle right now. That's a big claim, I know. I like making big claims and then aiming to prove them - and I haven't' finished yet! I hope I have actually exceeded your expectations, and again this isn't to impress you but so that you know what you're learning is the real deal. I want - I need - you to be confident in the skills because confidence in itself goes such a long way to being able to fight someone off. In fact a confident attitude has been proven as one of the most off-putting things for an attacker. If they think you are confident and they might have a difficult time dealing with you, they won't even try. So just from having these skills in your head means you might never get attacked. And then you'll be angry at me for making you go through all this and you never getting to test your skills!

So in the next twenty-thirty minutes, from now, of practice and understanding, you will make yourself quite unstrangleable. But if you do it today but never practice again and come back to me in a few years to say you got strangled…don't blame me - you have to review these skills regularly! I think they're as important as CPR and exactly like CPR you hope to never have to use them but have them in your skin and bones when you do. So come back and go through this book again, okay!

Let's get to chokes and strangles and, more importantly, how to beat them.

So, to be strangled or choked you need to have something pressing into specific parts of your neck or something wrapped around your whole neck. The wrapping can be anything really, from an arm to a thin scarf or it could be any chord in your room, like the phone charging wire or the tv one.

But for this action to be effective it has to go to the correct area of the neck to either squeeze the carotid arteries at the side and stop blood flowing from/to the brain, or it needs to be a squeeze of the windpipe to stop air from going in or out of the lungs.

As you've just worked out, if you didn't know before, a choke is when the airflow is stopped and the strangle is when the bloodflow is stopped. The differences between these two are mostly arbitrary for our purposes.

So to choke you, they would have to apply pressure to your windpipe and to strangle you they have to apply pressure to the big arteries, which are at either side of your neck.

I'm going to call both these things chokes from now on as it's just simpler and anyway, often it doesn't matter if someone is strangling or choking because the defences work for both. If I need to differentiate then I will do that but generally I will refer to the whole thing as chokes.

What we are going to deal with is this position here.

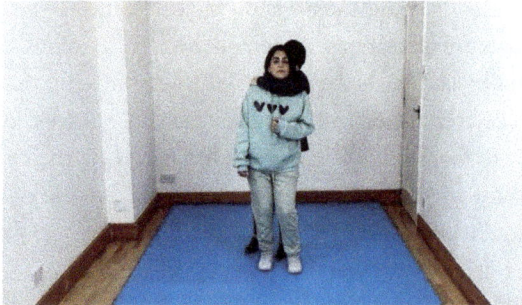

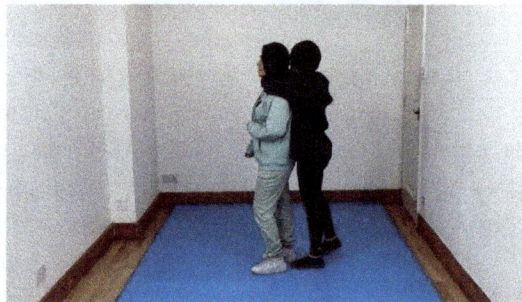

Although we are dealing with the standing up version of this, the same principles apply if you were on the ground and someone was going to choke you from behind.

So let's keep this really easy. The very first thing you have to understand is that this only works, and a choke can only be applied, if you are exactly where you are in the photos above. In other words the back of your head has to be in a set area for them to be able to get an arm around you to choke! Very few instructors seem to know this for some reason, yet it is so obvious, isn't it?!

So you must be in the square area as shown by my sister Rahilla below. If the Bad Guy is here you can choke him.

If you are here for the bad guy then you are in the choking area.

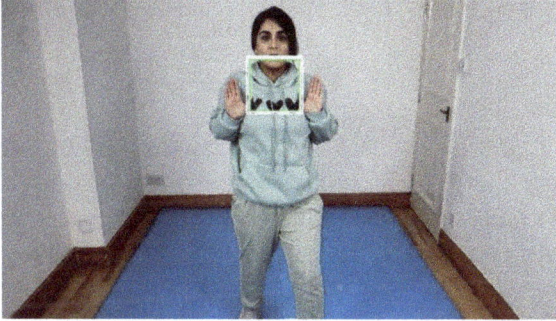

So, if you don't want to be choked then DON'T BE IN THAT SQUARE AREA! It is really quite that simple.

If you are lower or higher than that area…or to the left or right of it… then it is really quite difficult for him to choke you!

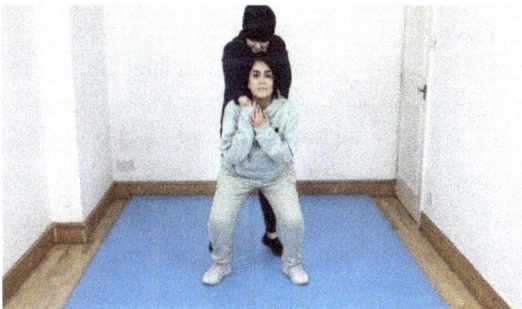

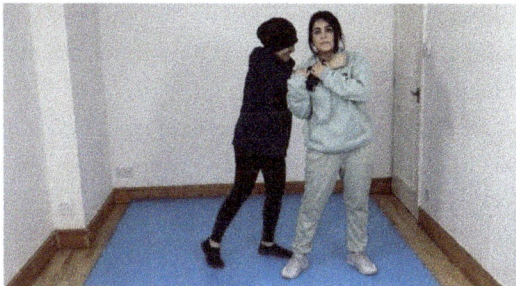

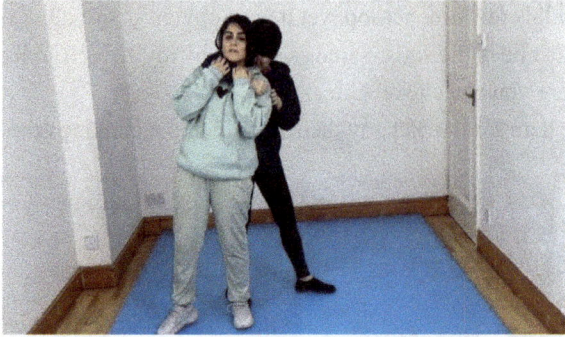

This is for demonstration purposes so not quite correct, but as you can see, moving off to the left and right or below the choke area renders the move unfeasible.

In reality Bad Guy will be fighting to keep you in position but should you be able to slip into these areas beyond the square, you are safe for the time being.

With regards to being higher than that square, this is usually possible when you're on the floor. If he is behind you when on the floor and strangling you, you can push upwards and go higher than that area.

So what we are dealing with here is avoidance. We are avoiding him getting to the right spot to start with . But avoidance starts much much earlier. You should't be waiting until he's got as arm around your neck. In martial arts classes and videos they teach how to get out of a full strangle, where someone has got their arm around your neck, secured it fully and now you try to escape. Yes, you do need to know how to get out of that too. But seriously, if someone was to do that to you right now, I very much doubt you'll get out. The choke is a serious position. The only place you're going next is unconsciousness or death. Those people who can escape a fully applied choke have already got a lot of serious skills under their belt and even they might not escape it. The choke is a check-mate position. And those who do escape it often have years, sometimes decades, of foundational skills they've practiced. That's why they can escape those deep full-on chokes. I don't know why they think that a layperson can also escape so easily. You can't. You might, but I doubt it.

And anyway, even if you have the skills to escape, are you going to wait until they've got a full choke when you could have avoided it and escaped it in so many ways before that? No! You still want to avoid first - and escape early if the avoidance did not work.

So we must avoid getting deep into the choke at all costs. It is an end-game move, as I have said. If you fail to get out of a deep choke, then your life is on the line.

To avoid and escape properly requires a good understanding of the methodology of the choke.

So to start with, the person will not have their arm around you. They might be far away like this.

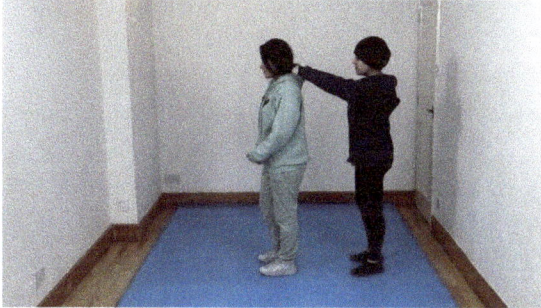

Now is the time for you to turn towards them.

They can't strangle you without the back of your head being at about their chest, therefore, facing them, at any time they try to strangle you, whether standing or on the ground, eliminates the choke attempt.

Read that again because it's worth half a kilo of ethically sourced Indian gold.

Of course in the above example you would move away, get The Fence up and start to fight him off should he grab or hit you etc. Please, remember that. But just for the moment we are focusing on dealing with chokes.

So, let's say you miss the early opportunity, next the attacker has to move in very close to you and pass their arm around over your shoulder, like this.

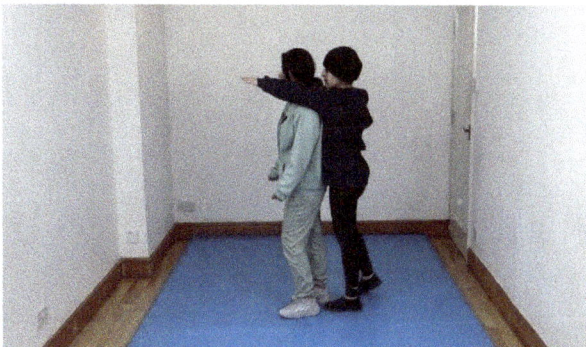

You are very likely to see and feel this arm coming over and in that case you can react to this. You may still be able to move away forwards. You may be able to turn into him quickly. You may still be able to duck lower or move to a side, quickly. You may also be able to take his arm as you do all that.

Let's say he's actually reached the next stage where he's got his arm around your neck area.

It's now going to be more difficult to move out of the square area at his chest and/or to turn your face towards him. But keep these in mind and do them as soon as you can.

So let's start with controlling his arm first. This is a man. He's likely to be strong as well as have strong intentions to get round your neck and stay there. So we have to stop that arm from being able to fully wrap around our necks.

So you need to take hold of his arm as shown, with your fingers curled over the top and pull his arm.

You may only be able to do this with one hand rather than both but make sure you are strongly pulling his arm and locking it where it is. Do not let it get secure around your neck.

You need to engage your lat muscles and pull down as well as your hands and arms.

You also need to make sure you have balance too, so that means - you guessed it - widening feet apart and dropping hips if possible. At least getting some kind of strong structure that you can work from, which will also counter him from dragging you away.

Something like this will do the job.

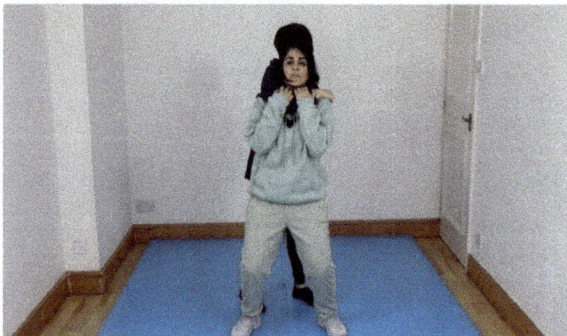

From here, while trying to peel his arm off, and pinning it to your body so he can't move it, you can potentially spin round to face him. The spin round will be towards the direction of his elbow.

Keep ducking lower and turning to him as you spin round.

So, if you are safe and under good supervision, have a go at all this. Get your training partner to go behind. And they slowly bring an arm round past your shoulders.

First just feel or hear their arm coming round. Quickly move around to face them before they can grab you. You may need to knock their arm out of the way, you may need to duck lower or move off to the side. You may be able to move forwards. Try all these things.

Next, if their arm has come round, quickly secure that arm to your body, and turn to face your partner. (Push them away, move away, get into the Fence, be ready to deal with anything else).

After a few repetitions, you can allow your partner to get their arm around a little more. No strangling, but maybe they can make the hold a little stronger. This time you'll need to make sure you secure that arm so it can't continue it's journey. Make sure you have balance as you hold on, and turn your body and head towards the elbow and escape out.

You are now starting to escape out of chokes. If you've had a few goes at that, let's make it an ever better defence.

So to choke you the arm needs to go around your neck.

Without your partner, on your own, I want you to tilt your head up and back. In other words lift your chin up high and move your head back so the distance between your chest and chin elongates.

After you've done that, I want you to tilt your chin down, towards your chest. Really make the distance between chin and chest as short as you can. Touch your chest with your chin.

Of those two positions you've just done, which do you think would be easier to get an arm around?

Of course, with your chin down there is less exposure of the neck. You've almost hidden your neck!

Now, as you duck your chin down, I want you to 'turtle' your neck in. Shrink your neck down into your body like you were a turtle AND shrug up your shoulders so they're touching your ears.

You have now reduced this area even further!

In this position ask your partner to put their arm around your neck. (Not tight at this time if you are just starting out in this type of training).
See how difficult it is for him to get around your neck?

So, actually as soon as you feel an arm is going to strangle you, you immediately move into this position with your head and shoulders. At the same time you move your hands up to hook his arm and you turn out so the back of your head is not touching the aforementioned square.
And you are now starting to become strangle-proof!

So you need to learn that. Practice it. The more time you give it the better prepared you will be able to deal with it. Just note that again this is not neat and tidy. This is a fight situation. You will sometimes miss the arms when you're in a rush. You will sometimes turn the wrong way. You will make mistakes. But there is enough there to really protect you with a little practice.
We're not finished yet by the way. So to actually strangle you requires particular things to happen. We've already covered the fact he needs to be behind you and the back of your head needs to be in the square area as shown, and he also needs to get his arm around your neck (which we've hopefully stopped by turtling etc) and then he has to squeeze that arm around you neck. So let's deal with this squeezing next.
So, to squeeze and cause you issues, he has to keep his arm tight around your neck. With his arm wrapped around your neck, like an evil scarf, he has to squeeze. If the arm is just doing that on its own it is not an easy task for him and he will be less successful than if he secured his arm and choked from there.
Below for example, where the circle is, is where his hand is actually grabbing onto your clothes so he can secure that arm. He might try to squeeze from here with just that arm, which could be effective but most likely it won't.

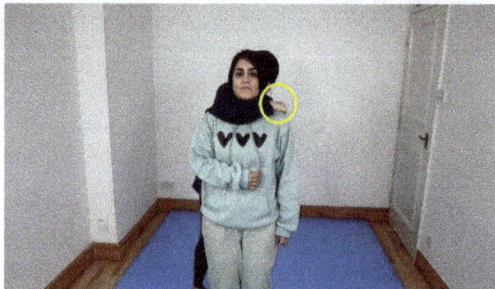

So he will secure that hand by grabbing it with his free hand (or he might use use some other technique to secure that hand so he can squeeze).

So our job here is to not let him squeeze and not let him secure that hand, whilst we continue to turtle and to duck down or to the sides and move the back of our head off the square area.

Simple!

I'm joking. It's not that simple, but with practice you'll make it automatic. There's actually not that much to do in reality but it comes with repetition.

So, in short:

you're going to avoid or get away from the square,

you're going to turtle your neck and shoulders, and

you're not going to let that arm/hand (with a yellow circle around it) get secure because you're going to hold or peel it off by grabbing it and pulling it down using your lat muscles.

Just three things. I hope that makes sense.

And with all that, you now have the ability to deal with someone choking you from behind.

This seriously works. It really does. If you're into martial arts and do jiu jitsu or wrestling or any other art where you can get choked from behind, try this, and you'll find you've become virtually un-strangle-able.

These skills above really will keep you out of trouble. But the fact remains that the choke is a very dangerous move. If someone gets the full position secured on you and knows how to apply it, or they're just using brute force at that time, then you're in deep trouble. There are some possibilities to deal with it but you're now entering into another territory that requires a decent amount of study. But I genuinely haven't been strangled in a very long time by using these above principles, against trained fighters who really knew how to choke and strangle.

So those are the direct methods of dealing with chokes. Indirectly you could go for eye pokes if you reach your hand over your shoulder, and use your thumb or fingers. You could also grab one or two of his fingers and immediately pull the arm off. You could go for his groin with one hand and I'm sure you can also come up with some other things you could try, such as biting his arm or scratching it if he is bare armed or wearing thinner clothing. You can even trip him or throw him if you have the skills to do that too.

Just one more point before we move on. There is the possibility even earlier to avoid this. For example, if you are being followed you should not be waiting until he starts putting an arm around your neck. You should have already acted prior to this. Read the chapter Man Approaching From Behind to assist you with a great strategy that I used hundreds of times to save me on the streets of London.

I'll see you in the next chapter.

WITH REGARD TO SEXUAL ASSAULTS, INCLUDING RAPE

With avoidance and with the skills you've already learned you should be many steps ahead of any attacker, whether their intentions are to sexually harm you or otherwise. You have created blocks and defences starting from his approach all the way to the Deep Fight area. The skills you have learned in the Deep Fight apply to and help deal with sexual assault too. But obviously there is always the chance to be caught off guard or he plays his game very well and we are now not in a great place and need to work our way out.

It could also be that you did not expect this to happen and it is all a surprise. There was no approach or anything else because this was a person you trusted up until that point. Sexual violence also takes place in domestic situations and so you might never get the chance to apply any of those early defences we have talked about and practiced. But this book is for everyone and I didn't want to firstly trigger emotions too strongly if I could help it and secondly I don't want younger girls to read things that are may be too much for them. I am not qualified in trauma areas and so I have no right to talk about is as if I am. (As I have mentioned before, you can go to www.power-for-women.org/complement).

But currently, all of the skills you have learned here also apply to any of the more serious situations. Everything in this book still applies and can be used to fight off these most heinous of people anyway so do keep that in mind.

MOMENTS OF POWER

When you watch a movie you will see moments when the bad guy has the power and then when it shifts to the Good Guy. In the final battle with the big Bad Guy, the Boss in some form or other, the power will shift back and forth between the Bad Guy and the Good Guy. This is actually how real life is, and maybe why this process works in films and novels.

Self defence is not just one continuous overwhelm. There will be pockets and places where actually you have the upper hand for a moment, and when he does. There is another time too, where neither of you has power. That's for example in the movie when the gun appears and it's two metres from both the good guy and the bad guy, and they both see it at the same time and they both jump and roll to get it. They both want the upper hand and they are pretty much equal at that time - and both have the potential to get the upper hand.

In real life, you might not be able to jump for a gun (or a knife or a brick) but there will be those times when the Bad Guy does not have power.

As a martial artist my aim is always to have power for as long as I can, but I am fully aware that I cannot have it all the time. Most of fighting, as every fighter will know, is about recovery and trying to regain power after losing it. It is not constantly dominating and dominating. The word 'fight' implies struggle. And that struggle is taking place even for the person who may appear to be winning right now. They might be winning for this moment, but you know what, it's because they are fighting and focused on the task at hand and keeping their struggle going. The second they lose focus or make a mistake, is the second their dominance can be challenged.

Even when I'm losing badly, and continuously, for a long while, I know it only takes one break for me to escape or to hit them or to do something that will gain me victory. I know that.

In fact if you watch any big fight competition, let's take the Ultimate Fighting Championships that I have been watching and analysing from when they were only available on bootleg video in the late 1990s. Often a fighter will be losing for 20 minutes, but he keeps going because he knows there will be a moment - and it will only be a moment - where he might be able to take advantage. In a very recent fight, between Leon Edwards and Kamaru Usman, the fight almost went the entire 5 rounds of 5 minutes each. Usman was beating Edwards down continuously and somehow Edwards held on for dear life. In the last few minutes of the fight, from what appeared to be nowhere, Edwards kicked Usman in the head and won the fight to become the new champion. Many viewers say he was lucky but I'm not too sure. I say it was skill and resilience. He had practiced that kick. It wasn't some random kick. And in a fight situation you sometimes only need that one chance to turn the whole thing around. I've seen this happen hundreds of times and so would you if you'd watched sports fighting for as long as I have.

Now, I'm not a fan of violence or watching it but I've been in it all my life and I study it still to this day. I watch the UFC's to see the skills of the fighters and their methodology and their tenacity. I also know I was headed in that same direction of competitive fighting at one point but it went against two things - one I don't like to hurt people for money and two it is not self defence, so was taking me away from the thing I needed in real life. Actually a third reason was that I also don't like to be slipping around on someone else's blood and getting it into my mouth and my cuts mixing with his cuts and blood being inside us and all over us. That's not my thing, although visually they have virtually sanitised all that now because they move the camera away from the major injuries and they're quick to wipe the fighters down with a towel between rounds, so you can't see they are dripping in blood head to toe. That could put people off from wanting to watch two men (and now women) smash each other for money. But I'm digressing again!

We were talking about moments of power. What you need to look out for are both psychological and/or physical drops in power. There will be moments when he has to move his attention onto something else, for example if it's a sexual assault then he has to do things to achieve his goals - has to remove clothes etc.

He can't multi-task, no human can. All we can do is switch between tasks and women are quicker and better at it than men. So as he hangs onto one task - keeping you to the floor for example - and moves to removing an item of clothing, he is now vulnerable as he is not focusing on the 'keeping you held down' as much. He is doing it on automatic but he is not focused on it. And there is a moment for you to fight back. There are many moments of shifting power like this.

One great way to become more aware of them is… Guess what?… Training and practising! So get on with it, please! As you feel what your training partner is doing, you will notice the times when they are distracted or when they move to do something else or when they take a breather, and there is your gap to escape or attack.

The point is that there are moments of power from the very beginning to the very end. Look out for them. They can change the entire situation to your advantage in a millisecond.

SOMETHING VICIOUS HIS WAY COMES

There will be times when you have to go a bit visceral, a bit animal, when you're in real danger and no way you're going to let him beat you. No way. No way is he going to damage or kill you.

Only you know if you are in real danger or not. Your brain will be telling you. It's a very good guide and the law should/will take into account what you believed to be true at the time.

My advice is that you don't override your brain. It's also the advice of Gavin DeBecker. DeBecker is the bodyguard of many people at the top of the economic and political food-chains, from presidents to celeb dynasties, like the Beckham empire and Oprah Winfrey.

When you are in deep danger, you have to survive. You are working at quite an intense level, right?

If you watch movies you might see someone who's life is in danger. They're very calm about their life being in danger. They'll go along with whatever they're told. They'll maybe be quite cerebral. Even those who fight back right away are usually quite controlled about it.

Now, this might be the case sometimes. It might be that you've watched a lot tv and somehow managed to copy that or it might be you're a trained person, so you don't do what the rest of us will do.

The rest of us will *literally* fight for our lives. Like, *literally*.

It means we will try everything. It means we won't let the guy tie us up all nicely and calmly like they do in the movies.

It means we will try to kick his face and the car window as he holds us down on the back seat.

It basically means we will do anything at that time. Because it might be the last time we actually ever do anything ever again.

This is a bit strong of a strong thing to ask you to do, but imagine if you genuinely believed this person was going to kill you. How would that feel? What are you willing to do, whilst in that state, to survive and get away?

So we're going to go over a few things here but the first thing is to understand the Bad Guy's thought processes.

If this person is fully committed to doing us harm, then in no way is he going to let on. It's just not likely. There are obviously going to be occasions when he does and we become aware early, and in those cases we can start acting early. Then we have the progressing situations, as you have seen in Stages One to Four, from the Early to the Deep.

But these people know we will fight back if we genuinely think our life is on the line. We're not going to just let him take it. It's not even our decision. The brain will override everything and fight for our life. He knows this. He doesn't want to spike your natural instincts to fight for your life because you're not going to be an easy target then, are you?

So guess what?

He will be trying to bypass your instincts all the time.

He only can do that in a few ways though.

He can be kind and polite and ensure you believe that he is a trustworthy and decent person, right up until he pounces.

He could also override you emotionally. He's got a gun or a knife. Or he's somehow mentally dominated you. You know you are in deep danger but there isn't much you can do about it right now. Any action that you take will get you killed. And so you are subdued by this knowledge. You go along or you die right there, you think.

Another way he can get us is to pounce really quickly before we can even get any chance or much of a chance to assess him or the situation. You could be hit over the head for example. You could be tied up rapidly before you even know it. You could be in a car and it gets locked.

In all these situations you will have to go animal at some point to save your life.

It might not even be these severe life-threatening situations. It could be anytime you realise your life or limb is genuinely in danger, then you should protect yourself.

So we really need to look at what can be really dangerous moves. Ways to really hurt or kill. I'm not going to cover too much of this as I don't want everything out there in the world for everyone to know, but I do want you to have some usable knowledge.

There are many ways to knock someone out, for example. Make them unconscious in other words. Some of these techniques you can learn only from a few masters who specialise in such things (and you have to have paid your dues in time and effort and money to access them, as it rightly should be. These are not techniques for everyone to know though as they won't be good in the wrong hands).

We're going to cover a bit of what you need to make you pretty darn dangerous but we're not going to turn you into assassins. We're going to continue with self defence rather than fighting skills.

Momentarily returning to the above situations where he's overridden your ability to go animal, you will have to wait for the moment when you can switch on the animal. In the Gavin DeBecker book *The Gift of Fear* there is a story of a lady who was tricked into letting a man carry her groceries into her flat. She was overloaded with them and he coerced her into carrying them into the flat, where he produced a gun. So she was controlled right away and she could not fight because otherwise she was going to be dead. The man did what he was going to do and then at one point, accidentally, he allowed the lady a moment to walk out of the room to go to the bathroom. She took that moment but instead of going to the bathroom she left through the front door and hid at a neighbour's and kept her life. She felt that the man had every intention of killing her. He was just working towards the right moment. It was that feeling, that instinct, that allowed her to walk out of the flat and survive. She was very brave to make that decision at that ultimate time of distress and walk out when he could have heard her open the door.

In this case there was probably never a moment when she could fight him and at the last minute she managed to just walk away. But if there was a chance then she would have had to go animal.

So I don't want to take away your instincts to survive. I don't necessarily say that you should or should not be cerebral at the time and think the situation through. Only you know what to do that at the time. What I want to do is just give you a few extra things that you could use in those most dangerous of situations.

You actually already know quite a few. So a decent snap-kick to his groin (driving up to his bellybutton) is going to help, as will a deep gouge into the eyes and some of the other things you've already covered. So don't lose track of what you've already learned. They will get you out of most situations. But I like to go an extra little mile so let's add just add one more layer to your ability.

UNCONSCIOUSNESS

So you may or may not have gone animal, gone visceral, but these targets and principles will work whether you have or haven't. It's just that they have quite strong effects so you don't want to be using them in minor situations.

We're going to start with an understanding of unconsciousness.

Here's the thing with unconsciousness; scientists can never find enough volunteers to let them whack 'em til they go to sleepy-byes. Apparently it might all be a bit unethical too. So the research on the actual process of how it happens is not vast to say the least. Much of it is anecdotal and some of it is theoretical. But as a martial artist who has studied this a lot and for a long time, I have hundreds and hundreds of recorded videos of people getting knocked out. (They're not for sitting down viewing of an evening though, chilling with tea and cake. They're actually quite nasty to watch but it's what I did.)

I've also read quite a lot about this and spoken to martial artists who know about such things, so that means you don't have to watch all those videos and you'll find out the necessary information from me! You can thank me later. I'll have some pistachio ice cream, thank you.

The very first thing you need to understand, so you can be effective right away, is that knocking someone out using blunt forces to the head area (such as Palm Heel, kick, baseball bat, brick, punch, elbow etc) can happen from one really hard shot or an accumulation of shots, or anywhere in between.

In other words, if you want to knock someone out, hit them in the head as hard as you can and as many times as you can until they go unconscious.

This could be anywhere on the head. It can be the top or the sides or it can be the front or back. Palm Heels and elbows are probably the two most accessible weapons to use for this, whether you're standing up on on the ground. You can use them to hit all areas of the head.

I want to remind you again, to make someone unconscious, you might do it via one big shot or an accumulation of many smaller shots. This is important for us to remember. If we can't hit someone really hard, maybe because we are being held too close to them and held tight, we can still cause concussion as long as we just keep hitting and hitting.

But always hit as hard as you can. If you are hitting someone then there must be a valid reason for it, I would guess. In that case you should hit them hard.

This brings us the next point. What we are actually trying to do is cause concussion here. For our purposes we need to understand that concussion is caused by brain shake or by the brain hitting the sides of the scull. The brain is actually contained in a sack of fluid in which it 'floats'. What we want to do is make that brain shake a lot and/or hit the sides of the scull on the inside. The brain doesn't like this very much and so it switches off to have a rest before it resets.

So when you are hitting to cause concussion, you need to hit deep into the head. Surface shots will not do the trick. We have covered this already that when you hit a target you hit right through. You're not hitting the head per se. You're trying to get right through and hit the brain to make it shake, rattle and roll.

Remember that you can hit the head with one of your own weapons or you can hit the head into something else, such as a wall or the ground. This is much harder to do and the chances of such a situation arising are smaller but it's worth knowing. If you can bang his head into a tree in the park, or the concrete floor of the multi-storey car park, or the door of the hotel room, just make sure you understand that it's not to cause surface damage to his head. It's to cause his brain to shake. So drive that head through so it comes out of the other side of the tree or door.

Sounds a bit violent but we've reached the Deep Fight for your life here and he's left you no option.

HIT HIM IN THE JAW

You may already know that a good whack to the jaw can cause unconsciousness. This is apparently because a hit to the jaw causes brain shake. The jaw is connected to the scull and a good shot at the jaw causes it to vibrate right up inside the head.

The jaw starts just under the ear, includes the chin and carries on to the other side, under the ear again. Have a check on yourself to see where it starts and finishes. Move your jaw and any part of it that moves is a target for you to hit.

In the boxing world it is said that it doesn't take much power to knock someone out if you catch them nicely on the jaw and if he doesn't expect it. This has been proven many times over. A good clip to the jaw does send people unconscious when they were not prepared for it.

So the perfect time to hit is when he's not expecting it.

This is especially applicable if you're doing a pre-emptive strikes. If he's talking, asking a question or answering, or even if he's thinking about something you just asked, you can catch him unawares with a good shot. This is often what happens in men's self defence. One guy will always attack the other when he's not ready for it.

As has already been said, you don't have to hit the jaw too hard, though you should hit it as hard as you can.

Hitting the jaw at angles is also a great thing but maybe a bit more of an advanced technique, but it does increase the chances of a knockout. The jaw is quite easy to break if hit at angles, and it really does hurt when that happens. It is major trauma and not just a bit of pain and so has potential stoppage power even if he is not unconscious. So don't think you have to hit the jaw square on. Just hit it as hard as you can and you should see some useful effects such as him letting go if he's grabbed you, or at the least you will distract him so that you can do something else for a second.

HIT HIM IN THE NECK

A good shot, or several shots, to the neck can really help your cause to escape and live.

You can hit pretty much anywhere on the neck to get decent effects. Again you should hit really hard, hit many times, and keep on hitting until you are safe. One shot might not do the trick, especially if he's got a thick neck or he's got a coat with a collar preventing you reaching the target properly.

The neck has several places you can hit. The entire throat is quite vulnerable. You might have seen karate chops used to hit that area in old movies. You could hit it with a punch or palm heel. You could press your knee onto it if you're on the ground in a top position. You could hit it with an object such as your mobile phone or an umbrella or a folder or whatever comes to hand at the time.

The neck is a vulnerable and painful area to hit. Remember that a shot there could be lethal.

Also remember that it might not be as easy to hit as you might think it is. During a fight you'll both be moving about so small targets are not always easy to get to. But should it present itself to you, like hors d'oeuvres on a tray at a party, you should get at it.

To one side of the throat is the area called the brachial plexus (coloured yellow in the diagram)

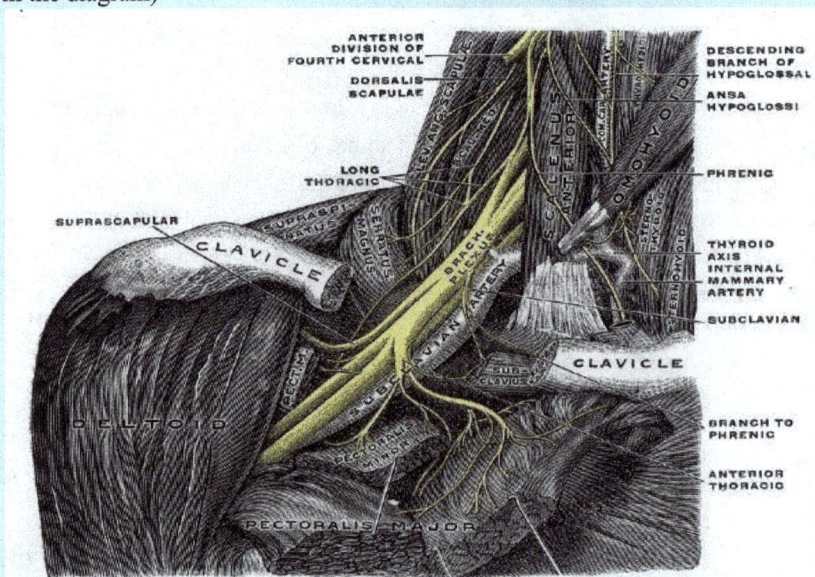

Hitting anywhere on this area sends strong signals to the brain. At least it will be a sudden sharp pain that he has to deal with. At best you will knock him out, in which case he will literally collapse like a building being demolished with explosives.

Again, hit many times rather than hit once then stand back and admire but one good shot in this area will drop him. If you can get to this area that is.

To find this area on yourself, get your thumb or index finger and press your clavicle in several places. You will feel a sudden pain when you press a nerve located at a spot there. This is the the bottom end of the brachial plexus. It then travels up the side of the neck and goes under the neck muscles, which is why you do need to hit this area quite hard, to hit through the neck muscles.

The brachial plexus is a really good target to aim for. Should you miss it, you might hit something else nearby anyway.

If we keep going round the neck, past the brachial area, we move to the side of the neck. There are plenty of nerves here too. Though they're smaller than the brachial plexus they're not protected by the thick neck muscles. So this is another area you can hit really hard and get a decent reaction from. This area is less likely to make him unconscious but some good solid hits here could get some useful effects. At the least you will cause reaction and pain. This pain is more like the toothache pain you get, when a nerve in the tooth is exposed to the air. This is a different and deeper pain than the one you can override by just using your mind.

If we continue around we get to the back of the neck. Here the cervical spine is near the surface and not very well protected. You can feel this area at the back of the neck. The bones you feel there at the back of your neck are the cervical spine. In most combat sports this area is not allowed to targeting but for us it is a valid target. Again blunt forces (Palm Heels, Karate chops, heavy objects) can be used here. You can usually access this area if the person is ducking below you or if you are behind them whether standing up or on the ground.

And that brings us to one of the most dangerous areas you can hit. The Occipital Protuberence.

It's not the protuberence you're probably thinking of! This one is on the scull.

HIT HIM IN THE OCCIPITAL PROTUBERANCE AND THE MASTOID

This is probably the most dangerous place you can hit anyone and so you should be wary of this. Depending on how you hit it and how hard, you could easily cause severe damage and death. For that reason I am not going to show you the proper techniques to hit this area but I am going to say that you can really hit it with anything and that will cause enough effect anyway for you to get away.

To have a feel of where this area is, place your index finger just below your ear, on you neck, just behind the jaw. That is kind-of the mastoid area. Now move your finger horizontally from here and all the way to the back of your neck. At the back of the neck if you go up a bit you'll feel there is a ridge. This goes all the way across the back of the head and is called the occipital protuberance.

Here's a picture to show you whereabouts it is.

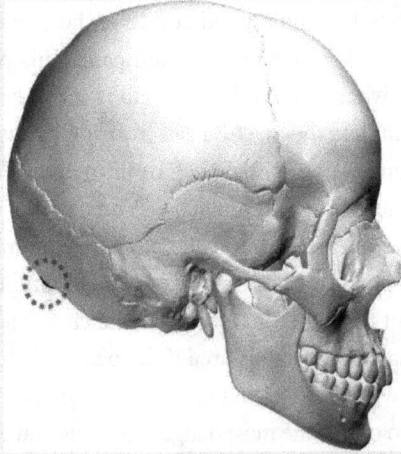

Just so you feel how this area is so effective, you can rap your knuckles all along it. In fact, try this (if no one is watching). Take your knuckles and then pat yourself with them anywhere on your head. The top or sides etc. Now do the exact same tap anywhere on the occipital ridge, using the same force. You should notice that hitting your head wasn't pleasant but hitting the occipital ridge did far more, like made your vision shake and suchlike. Hopefully you didn't do it too hard and ended up with a headache. But if you were to hit that area harder during a fight it multiplies that effect of wobbling the brain.

There's actually more going on in that area depending on how you hit it but for this book we're going to keep it basic.

Hitting Bad Guy at the back of the neck, anywhere really, will cause some serious effects. You can actually hit a little higher than the occipital ridge, hit the back of the head that is, and it will still be a very effective shot too.

So these areas all around the neck are pretty dangerous for the recipient. There are several ways to hit them that inflict different degrees of damage, but you have to study and practice them and some of them are really only for ninjas, soldiers and assassins. For our purposes, if we are in the Deep Fght, or at any time when we feel our life or limb are in danger, and we are given no option but to cause severe damage to stop the person, then we want to be hitting these areas really really hard. Hit what he gives you at the time. At the end of the day, it's us or them, and they shouldn't have put us in this situation to have to make the kind of decision that we are now having to make.

I hope this extra bit of knowledge has been helpful to you but I do want to remind you not to take this lightly. These last few bits of knowledge are quite powerful and dangerous. I tell them to you hesitantly because I feel I wouldn't be doing my duty if I didn't. And they are only for use in truly threatening situations. But only you can decide at the time what is truly threatening to you or not. That judgement has to be left to you. So judge quickly but wisely.

STAGE FIVE: THE AFTER

WHAT TO DO IMMEDIATELY IF YOU HAVE BEEN INVOLVED IN VIOLENCE AND/OR SEXUAL ASSAULT

CAUTION

Please note that this is all a guidance and in no way is it legal or medical advice of any kind. It is for guidance and educational purposes only. You should seek medical and legal advice, from a suitable and qualified person, including someone from the legal profession or the police, with regards to whether you should use this advice.

IF SOMETHING HAS HAPPENED

First, get safe.
You need to be somewhere safe.

Then you need to do a variety of things listed below if you can.

You will be in shock. Your brain will be all over the place. You will likely be shaking from the adrenaline still in your system that has kept you alive.

You might potentially admonish yourself or dislike yourself but try not to. The Bad Guy is always at fault. Not you. Regardless of what you might be thinking, this is true.

You may have made mistakes along the way, but that doesn't mean someone had the right to do what they did. They are in the wrong and not you.

WHAT TO DO AFTER AN INCIDENT

First get safe.
Next deal with injuries right away and get medical help asap.

You might need to deal with your own injuries. Hopefully you know some basic first aid that you can administer to yourself. Stop any bleeding first.

If you are safe and all major injuries (bleeds especially) are being dealt with, you can contact the authorities (the police or whoever has jurisdiction where you are). Contact a friend or someone who can support you emotionally.

Next preserve evidence if you can.

If there has been any physical contact, or you have fallen, or there is any confusion, you **must** seek medical help as soon as you can. It is highly important to do that.

In fact it is worth contacting medical help in every such instance. People have died when they haven't done this.

You won't be able to find all the injuries and damage yourself. You might not even have felt a punch or remembered exactly what happened and you are not in a good state to assess the scale of the damage. Only another person is best placed to do that.

Victims have reported being in minor altercations and said such things as 'I think I was punched but it doesn't really hurt' or said 'I was just pushed a bit' only to later be found to have severe and life-threatening injuries. If there has been physical contact then you need to get that checked.

So, get medical help.

This may be an ambulance or paramedics you have called. Or make your way to a medical facility, such as a hospital or doctor's surgery.

You can call them. You can walk to them or get transport to them.

Here's another thing, qualified medical staff will also record the physical and psychological state you are in and all will count as evidence if the situation ends up in court.

WHEN YOU CALL, THE EMERGENCY SERVICES THEY WILL WANT TO KNOW:

Where you are right now

What injuries you may have and their severity

What happened

WITH REGARD TO APPREHENDING THE PERPETRATOR

In police investigations there is what is called The Golden Hour(s) Principle. This says that the actions taken and the responses within the first hour(s) will create the most evidence gathering opportunities, the ability to fast track urgent enquiries and prevent the potential loss of important evidence.

It can also lead to the suspect being apprehended much quicker and also a greater chance of them being charged and convicted. So please do try, if possible, to contact the emergency services asap.

This is all the guidance I can really give you without moving into police work and affecting the legal system therefore I must stop there.

So, in brief, get safe, seek medical assistance, contact the authorities and contact support. The highest importance is your health and well-being so make sure those are attended to first.

Take a snapshot of the above and save it to your phone ,somewhere easily accessible in times of emergency. You could include other emergency numbers and suchlike too.

For various helpline numbers for support after any attack please see the chapter on Helpful Resources or conduct an online search. But do always consider these organisations. I have worked with them many times and they are mostly highly professional, experienced and understanding of your needs at that time and very helpful. You can often call them anonymously and they won't pressure you to pursue court cases etcetera so they are worthy of a call in your time of need.

PART FOUR:
SOME SITUATIONS THAT
MIGHT WORRY
YOU

These are situations that might concern you more specifically. Things you might think about so I just wanted to cover them individually. You already have the skills to deal with these really but let's make sure your knowledge is complete because it is knowledge that will let you stay one step ahead and it will be knowledge that will beat him at the game that he starts.

THE LOCKED ROOM SCENARIO

By locked-room scenario I'm including all scenarios where you can't leave, where you must stay to finish the job. There may or may not actually be a locked room This could occur in the middle of the park where you can't run away and leave behind the child that is with you or any other situation where you're trapped physically or psychologically.

When you just can't leave.

This is a rare scenario but truly frightening for most of us. You will be at maximum fear as you feel there is no way out and you must fight and in that fight you must win. And so the pressure is on.

This is the area most martial artists train for but then never test their skills because it's just a rare occurrence. The difference the martial artist doesn't quite get is that now there is no referee and when you land on the floor, it won't be a beautiful landing on a springy floor mat. And this Bad Guy doesn't care for rules nor follow those that you've got stuck inside your head from decades of obedience to them. But we're not here to discuss martial arts.

So the 'locked-room' scenario is dangerous.

The most important thing for you here is focus. Fear will be overwhelming your whole system and if he's played his game correctly then he's managed to get you really scared and probably stopped you from taking action.

So the first thing is to remember what fear is. It is your body preparing to make you superhuman.

Thank you body!

Do you also remember how to increase focus on the task at hand?

Anger.

Now is the time to summon it. Now you really will go animal, but in a controlled manner, when the time is right.

His job is to keep you scared and to keep you fearful of what will happen. He wants you to know and feel that you have been over-powered by someone who is impossible to beat.

In other words he does not want you to focus on fighting back.

Here's something you must understand about this situation:
you have all the skills to deal with it.

It is in this kind of situation where The Magic Five will help you rise to another level. Having added only one of them to your technical skillset will enhance your abilities massively. Adding more than one will raise your levels even further. So make sure you have trained at the basic skills and then add The Magic Five to enhance everything.

The reality is that what you've learned so far is enough to really deal with anyone. Just because the room is locked doesn't devalue the skills you have learned so far. It just means you have to be ready to fight for longer and harder. Expect more ups and downs.

But the whole situation could just finish very quickly too.

Just remember that this is a more mental game now.

Remember he will be aggressive, dominate you, and try everything he can.

But he's just a man. And you know how to hurt one of those, make them unconscious, or worse if you have to.

You really do have to use everything you know, from trickery to physical skills. You know the ground game, you know the standing game. You know how to hit him in a variety of ways. You know how to send him to bye-byes.

If he's got you trapped, feign weakness, feign submission, then hit him when he least expects it.

Take your moments.

The locked-room scenario is rare. You've got the skills to deal with it. The only difference you might have to deploy every one of those skills to get you out.

But on the other hand, it might only take one of them. It might be the next one that you use.

So get angry, keep breathing and use everything you've got.

A TIGHT SPACE: INSIDE A CAR
(OR OTHER VEHICLE)

Assaults in vehicles occur a lot in the United States but they're not as frequent in the UK, luckily. When an attack actually occurs inside a car it is usually a partner, current or ex. A stranger attacking you inside the car is less likely unless you're ferrying random people about. The other way it could occur is if you are bundled in while getting in or out of your car. Someone forces you inside in other words.

The car is a good place if you can get in and lock it, leaving him outside. The side windows are nowhere near as easy to smash as most people think. I know because I've seen cops trying to smash through them hundreds of times. So it's unlikely his first few blows will break the window.

The same applies if you're trying to escape from the inside too, unfortunately. You're just not very likely to be able to kick the windows out. But you should always try as it will make noise and you can be seen from the outside, which you can't if you're lying flat on the seats.

What happens in a car or tight space is that you're obstructed. Walls and suchlike block your movement - but they also block his too.

It's claustrophobic and you're trapped.

If you get underneath him it's not going to be so easy getting out using just technique. Having a well developed Sensitivity (one of The Magic Five we have discussed before) will allow you to feel where he is. A good understanding of Body Mechanics will also enhance all your abilities. Palm Heels and other strikes will work well but really the more visceral attacks will work best. Something vicious has to flow towards him. It's time to poke and bite whatever you can, using the Kino Mutai method of holding it and ripping off whole areas repeatedly. It's not time for being squeamish, I'm afraid.

To escape from underneath you really need to feel where his weight is or where you are located and from there you can slip and slide out. You might be able to move in the direction of your head, or off to the sides, to slip away from him. You might be able to sit up too. That mid-position in the Get Up when you have your arm down can be used to create a frame from where you can rise upwards.

If you're on top then you have the chance to hit a lot and do all the visceral things too, probably as a priority, but as secondary attacks you have all the ways to send him unconscious and possibly the chance to hit him as much as you can and as hard as you can. But you can only hit what he gives you to hit. Personally,

I'd go animal first and foremost, even if I'm hitting, I'm just distracting him so I can get to the vital bits to do maximal damage and get away.

If you open a window in the car then do so as you can shout and be heard.

If only the child-lock has been used to lock the rear doors then there is a chance you can reach out and open the door from the outside. You can't open a door from the inside with child-lock on but you can from the outside (if central locking isn't activated).

The tight space is dangerous and scrappy and scary. Just try to breath, slide out and get on top if you can.

Remember that it is also tight for him too. He's also in that same space as you are and restricted in what he can do.

So if you're in any confined space, stay above him to start with. Should you find yourself underneath then try to work your way to the top (go in any direction that you can to achieve this) and commit to doing enough severe damage that he has to stop.

Just remember that all the skills you have learned so far can be adapted to this situation. There are only a few ways he can be on top or you can be on top. There are only a few things he can do or you can do. It's just that this is more scary due to it being in such a tight and claustrophobic space. But just as some of your movement is restricted, so is his.

The fact is that in the UK you are not all that likely to be attacked in a car or bundled into a van. It's something very scary to imagine happening but I bet you've never met a single person that it's happened to. The stats show it is a very rare occurrence. So don't fear it but do prepare for it just because you'll feel better knowing you can deal with it, especially when you go on holiday abroad where it happens a bit more.

MAN APPROACHING FROM BEHIND

A man is following you. Or you just heard someone behind. You're on the street on your own.

What are you going to do?

Here's a tactic you're definitely not going to find anywhere else because I developed it and I'm even more proud to share it with you because I know how effective it is. It has saved my limbs and life on a lot of occasions.

When men fight men, they face each other. They approach each other from the front more than 90% of the time. It's an ego thing . For women it's not like that. Women get approached from the rear a lot. They get followed or they are just ambushed from the rear.

Part of the reason why women are successfully attacked from the rear is that women don't know what to do when being followed. There is no strategy out there to help with this. The whole martial arts and self defence world doesn't deal with a man who is following you. They work on the martial arts principle of starting a fight facing each other, then staying to fight, man-to-man. Take him to the floor and fight till you choke him is the current vogue.

So if a man is following you, what should you do? Should you turn and face him? Should you challenge him

? What if he was just silly and unaware that he was following you and scaring you? (Even I've done that by accident!). Wouldn't it be silly to react when all he was doing was walking home and was never a threat? You'd look silly, wouldn't you?

In a real situation there will be many questions going through your head when a man is walking behind you, and they will all be at the same time, and they will all be confusing you and by the time you decide what to do you might already be in a confrontation.

So you must have a strategy, and be ready to apply it for every situation where a man is approaching you from behind . Because if you don't then there is the possibility that you will be grabbed and dragged away and it only took a second to happen.

From my experience of reporting hundreds of assaults, 1 believe that many women are not 'ambushed' as such but the attack comes across as if it was an ambush due to not taking the right action early enough.

(Not the fault of the 'victim'. The perp is always at fault, as I truly believe and have said many times).

Without taking early action, you are starting several steps behind and it will take considerable effort to catch up.

The thing is that usually before an attack, there is a period of time when the victim knows there is someone behind. This period might be very short, the person is only a few steps away, or it can be much longer and women can even be followed for many minutes. This is what usually happens more so than ambush attacks, which we will cover in the next short chapter.

So we have to have a strategy to deal with this.

As a police officer in the centre of London, or any town for that matter, you arrive at dangerous stations all the time. There are people stabbed and beaten, and it's a war zone. (Yes, you never see this because it's
usually cleaned up by the time you go through it in the daytime).

So when you arrive, you don't know who the good guys are or the bad and you don't know who's going to turn round and start on you. Everyone's drunk and some of them are fuelled up on freely flowing cocaine.

You don't know who's behind you or around the next corner or hiding under a car with a knife they just stabbed someone with. On top of that you've got fifteen drunk idiots, who are also often called 'members of the public'. These MOPs stop right now and they're gawping. They might encourage the others to fight each other or even fight you. It's free entertainment for them.

So there are people all around. Three hundred and sixty degrees. Surrounding you.

But who's going to harm you and who's not? You just don't know.

So I would stop, with my back against a safe place - a vehicle or a wall usually - and observe what was going on for a few seconds before jumping in. If someone's life was in danger then I often didn't have that luxury
and had to just dive in and hope no one hit me from behind, but more often than not you could spare a second or two. So I used this tactic all the time and I know it saved me a lot of nightmares.

Arrive at a scene, make sure my back was protected and then observe before making a move.

To this I would also add The Fence. A Covert Fence if someone approached me and wasn't a threat, but I would often deploy an Overt Fence too if someone approached quickly and I had to tell them to stay back.

I'm sure this is a tactic all police officers use although it's not something they are trained in. I used it throughout my whole police career.

But this isn't the full tactic I'm going to tell you.

One day a very bright senior officer figured out that he could cover a wider area and reduce officer numbers if he made us all patrol alone. He had orders from the government to reduce police numbers and if he did

then he'd get a promotion and a bigger pension for it. So he did exactly that. He didn't care if we lived or died or how dangerous it was. His promotion was far more important.

So we went on a strict diet of patrolling on our own. Day and night. On your own. If you crossed paths with another officer you genuinely had to be careful if you were spotted and reported for it. You literally had to account for it and make a note of any encounters with other officers in your notebook providing a reason why you were with another officer and for how long.

This is not a joke. It sounds like a dystopian nightmare filmed by Francis Truffaut but I am not making this up. It really was like that, very strict, for well over a year before it eased up a little but not a lot. Officers just found ways around it, to beat the system over time.

So I found myself walking the back streets of London, through dark nights, alone for that year.

Here's the thing - you probably weren't aware that police officers were forced to patrol alone. But *every* criminal and lowlife in London knew about it. It's their job to know such things. And so officers were beaten. One I know personally was beaten unconscious. But he got himself a nice job in CID rather than raising a complaint about it. Other officers got smacked but it was 'their own fault' for not conducting the correct risk assessment.

So criminals loved it and took great advantage of this.

I found myself in this scary, dangerous environment. Beyond that we were short staffed because so many officers were moved to locations far and wide to cover the severe shortfalls. There was literally not a single team I knew of that had the required number of officers. They would all have failed risk assessments so none were ever done properly.

Everyone was overworked and many were going off sick. Which meant in turn there were even less officers. You could walk around all night and not cross paths with any other officer for hours. I'm not exaggerating.

So I was patrolling the Harrow Road and Maida Vale areas at night on my own, knowing I was a solid five minutes away from a police officer coming to my aid if I screamed down my radio. That's a long time when you're being beaten.

I always walked around with my expandable baton out, which is a useless piece of equipment against real criminals but it looks dependable to tourists in London, right? (Luckily I'd done some Escrima stick- fighting and the Fiarbairn method and so was reasonably handy with that stick if I needed to be).

I'd walk along, past various notorious estates in London, which

you didn't visit unless you were accompanied by the riot police, that I was now walking past day and night on my own.

This is where my method was honed. If someone followed me I did this.

Basically I did not want anyone behind me getting the upper hand. Quite literally getting a hand round my head or neck or hitting me from behind or anything else.

So what did I do?

Just turn so that I could deal with them face to face. But not everyone was a criminal out to get me, right? So when I turned, I did it in a casual manner, and created enough space in front to allow them the opportunity to walk by.

So I'd be walking along the road, Maida Vale let's say, which was eerily quiet at night but also frequented by many drunks. On the east side of it are the houses of television executives and people who can spend upwards of £5million a house. The highly affluent St John's Wood area is that way too. But on the west side of the same road are council estates all the way along, piled one on top of the other, like giant blocks of Lego that's never been cleaned.

The road was always under-lit with very few street lamps, and there are hundreds of places that would make great hiding places for someone to jump out at you or suddenly appear a metre behind. These mostly were people just leaving their homes but police were also quite disliked in that area so you had to stay wary. I just couldn't have people walking behind me.

So when I heard someone behind me I would slide across to the nearest safe location, for example I'd move so my back was up against a wall and I would turn so that I would be facing the person, but not actually looking at them or engaging. I wasn't actually facing them but just facing in that general direction, with my Covert Fence up, until they had gone by and I knew I was safe to move on.

So that was it.

I had to deal with some incidents whilst doing this but most of the time I did not. Whether the person behind me was a threat or not was not something for me to consider. I just had a strategy and I employed it as soon as someone was behind me.

And I know this saved me from injuries and assaults many time. Those few incidents that I did have to deal with, one very scary one actually, meant that I was already facing the person and not starting on my back foot.

So in brief, in case you didn't get it:

Someone is approaching you from behind.

You move off to the side in a safe way, create your Fence, and allow them to pass. Hopefully that's enough, and you can go on your way.

Should he not pass by but decide to engage you in conversation, you deal with the early interaction, cutting it all short, and hopefully that is enough and he leaves you.

Let's say he's one of the rare breed who decides to attack after this interaction, or even before the interaction. You are already in The Fence and know what to do from here if he goes to grab you or hit you.

Doing this is not going to give the Bad Guy the chance to catch up and jump us from behind. That's the idea. And this tactic really works. You've got the skills for it, you just need to have a go at it yourself a few times.

AMBUSH ATTACKS

What can you do if you get ambushed?

Firstly, what is an ambush and how likely is it?

I've dealt several times with women who have been ambushed but a pure ambush attack seems to be quite rare. Usually when I've spoken to the 'victim' for a short time I've discovered that they had noticed this person but did not act on it. It might have been they only noticed him behind them a second before and didn't know what to do. It appears that many 'ambush' attacks were actually someone approaching from behind.

Ambushes do happen though. Of course someone could jump out and grab us, or maybe we were so engrossed in our own world that we didn't spot them until that very last second and now we are ambushed. We have stresses and and excitements and a life to live. We can't live life on our tiptoes waiting for a Bad Guy to attack us all the time.

But if you are ambushed, the man has the advantage to start with. He knows what he is doing. He knows the location. He knows where to hide. He knows when to jump out to get maximum effect so you are left vulnerable for the moment and he has the upper hand for that time.

So when you are ambushed you are basically jumping into the Deep Fight right away. You will either fight back immediately or you might freeze. The adrenaline rush will be massive and that will lead to massive fear. It may be that he does manage to control your body movements and that just adds to the fear.

The first thing is that you must get your brain under control.

But I think you know that I'm about to say. You have the skills psychologically and physically to deal with this guy. You need to focus, so to do that get angry and then go animal. He needs to regret making this bad decision today. And I have to leave it to you to make sure that he does regret it. I would love to be there with you in person but I won't be. But maybe my words will be.

In an ambush attack, you need to get angry and visceral. He's going to hurt you. He's going to take things from you that you really don't want him to take.

You could end up on the floor much quicker in an ambush because you were not ready. But here in this situation is where the training of Balance (we're going to do it in the next Part) is going to stop you from falling and help you get stability so you can fight back. Sensitivity and understanding of the

Centre of Mass is going to change everything that is going on. You're going to be able to push better and resist more. It is in these kinds of situations where you will really need to employ all your skills, preferably at an enhanced level. Which is exactly what The Magic Five do. So let's go there next and see what they do, shall we?

PART FIVE:
SELF DEFENCE MASTERY

So far you've learned quite a lot. I hope you realise that you really can take on someone who's bigger and stronger and get away from them, even if they have malicious intent. I hope you've realised that these skills are masterful and that you can use them at any time and any place. I also hope you can see how at every step of the way we have tried to avoid first and then have continuously tried to thwart his attack and stop him before he can progress further.

We have placed stumbling blocks in front of him at every step he takes or every move he makes but we have also prepared to deal with the worst situations too, the ones we aren't very likely to encounter but we do fear the most.

If we can't get away from him, then more fool him because he won't expect the onslaught and your ability and mindset to deal with him, harm him and hurt him.

But that's not enough! I won't be satisfied until I can take you to another level! I didn't spend all that time and effort training and learning and figuring things out so I could just store the information in my head! I need to get it out and into the world and share it!

So the next step is to enhance all those skills you already have. We are going to rise several more levels yet.

We are going have a play with what I call 'The Magic Five'. These are the five master skills that individually raise your game. Each of these has the ability to make you stronger in everything that you do.

That's a big claim, isn't it? Here I go again making big claims! This is probably the biggest of them so far.

"Each of these? Is going to make *everything* I do much stronger?" I hear you say.

Well, yeah. That's what I said. Okay, I'll tone it down a notch. It won't make everything stronger but it will seriously make most things (seriously, almost everything!) stronger.

One of the things that I set out to do and something that I pride myself on is my knowledge of universal principles of sport.

What are the principles that apply across all sports and can they be applied to self defence?

This was not a question I asked consciously but having done so many sports throughout my life certain things became obvious to me. I like being active. I always have. So I've coached and taken part in loads, from canoeing and sailing to racquet sports, rock climbing, gymnastics and a whole heap more. I worked at a gym in Hammersmith where I was lucky enough to coach various professional rugby players, some athletes and even ballet dancers from the Hammersmith ballet school. I've also coached visually impaired people and those with physical impairments. Coaching sports was also part of my degree programme and prior to that I completed a two-year coaching programme when I was doing A-Levels. Even before that, in the Royal Air Force Air Cadets I was coaching subjects such as rifle shooting, Duke of Edinburgh award and drill (marching).

So I've coached a lot in my time you could say, and I've also been into martial arts, you might have noticed.

What I discovered through all this was that there are performance enhancing principles that apply in almost every sport including the martial arts and self defence. And now it's your turn to find out about them. I hope you will practice them!

I would normally teach The Magic Five at the beginning of everything. In our two comprehensive Power For Women courses - the Foundations of Women's Self defence and the Complete Women's Self defence courses - these are the first things you would learn because they apply to so many things that you do afterwards.By doing it that way we automatically include them into every technique you learn from then onwards and so your skills are enhanced right away.

You've gone through most of this book now so knowing them will mean you already know the skills you're going to apply them to. They can literally be applied to everything you've done in this book so far.

They are the shortcut to being powerful. The shortcut to success out there in a world where you might need to use self defence techniques. Imagine knowing all the best skills out there - which you do already - and then adding these to them.

It's really something.

Knowing these will improve any sport that you take part in too - and you can even use them in daily life! But that's all past the scope of this book.

So let's get on and learn them!

Welcome to The Magic Five.

I can't wait to share them with you.

BALANCE

Balance. Base. Stability. These names are often synonyms in self defence to mean the same things but call it what you like. You need to understand it.

Having good balance, more importantly the ability to maintain good balance, will be what prevents you from falling, from hitting the floor. That's quite obvious to you now.

From a standing fight point of view it's about staying in balance so you can't be taken to the ground or dragged away or pushed somewhere you don't want to go. It also means that you can move around and away from danger. If your back is towards a busy dangerous road and his back is to a safe place, then you want to be switching sides. Make his back be towards the road or river or edge of the cliff while you move to the safer place. Let him fall to danger if he kicks off or when you push him.

To do this takes skill and knowledge, or luck, but you'll do better if you can keep good balance throughout.

Whilst standing if we are being moved around, then we can get that balance by having the correct footwork and by having a good base, both of which give us good stability.

Base, we can say, is having our feet correct for what we are trying to do. We go from the regular Fence to the Wide Fence for example when someone pushes or pulls us. We have just widened our base, so that we can be more stable right? And we moved our feet using good footwork to get there.

I hope this is all making sense. We are going to have a practice in a moment anyway.

The Australian John Danaher is a man I doubt you've ever heard of but he's considered the greatest working jiu jitsu coach in the world today. That's quite an accolade when you consider how many coaches there are in one of the fastest growing combat sports ever. In his words the first thing that your opponent requires is balance. If you can defeat his balance he is always on his 'back foot', he says.

The same applies the other way round too. If your balance is shot you are going to be a step behind, literally and metaphorically as well as mentally. It's not nice being shook around and not being able to get your footing. In fact, with bad footing you can hardly do anything. You can't hit, you can't move and you can't fight back or even get away.

But with good balance you are going to hit harder and do everything much better.

But I don't want to make your balance good. I want to make it great!

But you see, doing footwork, for most people, is one of the most boring things that's ever been invented. I am hoping that you'll go ahead and practice a lot. But I have my doubts so I'm going to say a couple more things about it.

I haven't mentioned Rickson Gracie for a while so let's bring him back into the conversation. Often considered the greatest street fighter in the modern world, he his also a true devotee to the fighting arts. One of those people who is so entrenched into martial arts that it's difficult to figure out if he is martial arts or if martial arts is he. Rickson has something he calls 'Base' as one of his five major principles of fighting and self defence. His five are not the same as my Magic Five in case you're wondering, and actually it made me laugh when I found out he also had five principles, and that one of them was exactly the same as I had! My first thought was that everyone will say I copied him but I really didn't! Anyway, he says that without 'base' you have a lot of weakness in everything you do. One of the first things he gets his students to work on is 'base'.

I'm going to mention one more coaching great - the late, great, humanist and boxing coach Brendan Ingle, whose boxing gym in Sheffield I trained in a few times back in the day. My youngest brother, Naveed, who is helping edit this book, was a regular and is a family friend of the Ingles.

Brendan made you spend months doing footwork when you first arrived at his gym. Literally months. He didn't even let you throw one punch until you'd done your time and showed your skills in footwork. Brendan

is a legend in the boxing world and a mentor to so many kids during his lifetime. He crafted several world boxing champions too, including Prince Naseem Hamed and Johnny Nelson you may have heard of.

So I know some of you might lose the will to live when you practice footwork/balance but please do it!

I've done my time with it. I used to put the tv on and walk about doing footwork for an hour. I used to do 'footwork' as I walked around the house. I just fitted it in to so many places, so maybe that is the way for you to do it too.

I'm not going to beg you anymore, but I'm just going to repeat that balance will determine how much power you can generate, how hard you can hit or pull or push, and it will help you to stay on your feet. One final thing, having good balance and footwork is something that will take you into old age. We lose balance as we age and practising it (via yoga if not from footwork drills) has been proven to increase it's longevity. So that's just one more reason to do it! Practice balance drills and you will keep your balance for ever!

Let's have a go, before you throw this book at me.

So, please, get into the Overt Fence position. From there you are going to move forwards first.

So your feet are in the square shape that we will always aim to maintain. From there, take a step forward with your front foot. And then catch up with your back foot to make a square shape again with your stance.

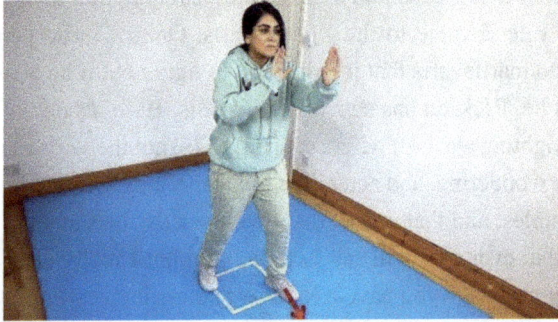

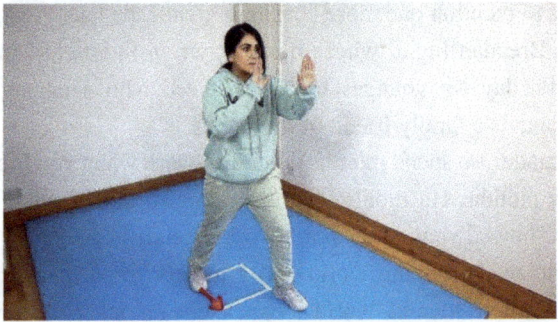

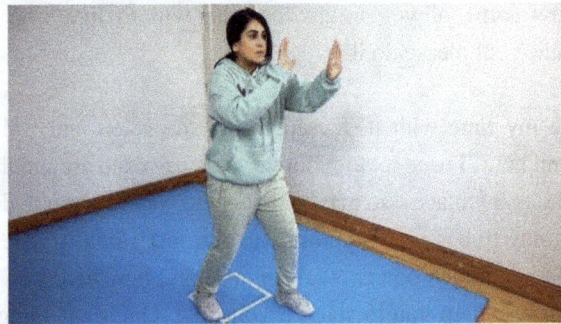

And that's it if you want to walk forwards!

You just repeat that again and again and you will keep going forwards until you hit a wall or fall into the sea or something.

Let's go backwards.

Starting in The Fence, feet square, knees bent, light on your toes (but heels are not off the ground), arms up…now take a step back with your back foot. And then catch up with your other foot so you are back into the square again. To move further back, do that again and keep going.

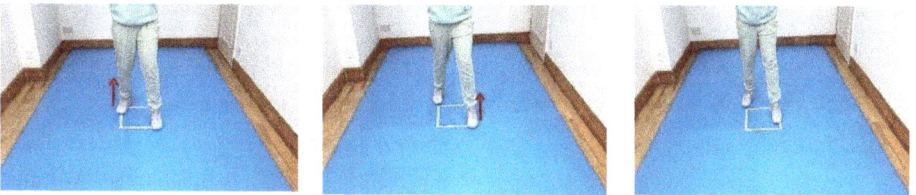

To move to the left you move first your left foot in that direction and then catch up with the other foot. Just a note to remind you to not take too big a step as you will then be off balance and defeat the purpose. If you need to move more than one step distance then just take another step. Simple!

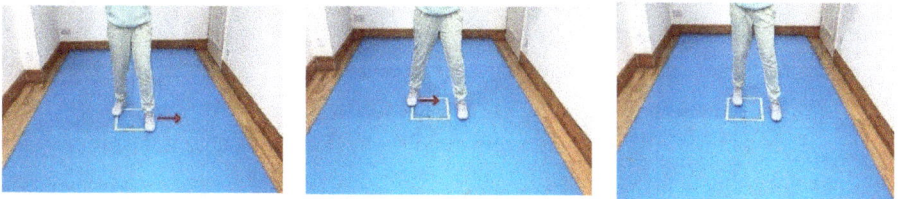

So to move to the right, move your right foot to the right and then catch up. As shown below.

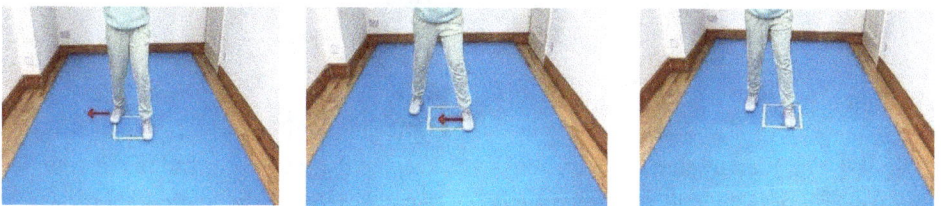

And that is it! You are now able to move in all four directions effectively.

Did you notice that to move forwards you moved your front foot; to move backwards you first moved your back foot; to move left or right you moved that foot first?

So this is the case even if you are a left-handed person. You lefties might prefer to have your right foot forward in The Fence, but for movement purposes it does not matter. You always move the foot first that is in the direction you will head to. So even if you find yourself not standing in the perfect Fence position because you've been pushed or you slipped or you're on grass or you have one foot on the pavement or one foot on the road, it doesn't matter. To travel left move your left foot, and so on.

So it is good to practice this slowly at first and then add some speed to it. Move quicker. Walk a few steps forwards and a few back. A few to the left and a few to the right.

Next, get your partner to pressure you a little bit. Get them standing in front and as they move towards you, you have to step back, and as they move back, you catch up with them. If they move left or right you mirror them! This can be a good fun game and a more interesting way to learn footwork too. But you can do this on your own and use your imagination if you want to practice but no one is around. You'll see boxers doing exactly that, for hours on end in the boxing gym, boxing their shadows.

But you can't just go back and forth and left and right. We're not robots. Sometimes we have to move out of the way if we get charged at or it might be that we want to move at angles for other reasons. In that case we need to also learn to pivot.

So starting with The Fence, this time we have drawn a dot on the ground and we are going to pivot around it.

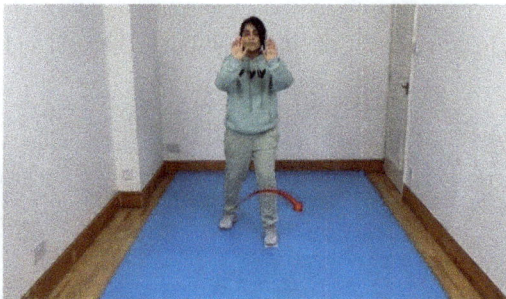

You literally turn on your front foot (keeping it where it is), and move your other foot in a circle. It might take you a few goes to get right but your aim is to travel about 90 degrees each time. This way you can be out of the way if for example if someone pushed you or charges at you (and you can let them fall into the road rather than you).

So from The Fence, pivot on your front foot to get into this position.

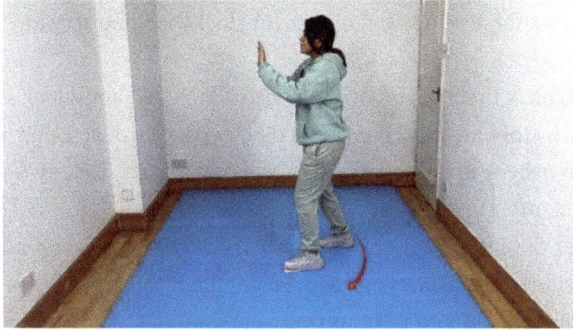

If you did the same move once more, you will be facing the opposite direction to the one you originally started in.

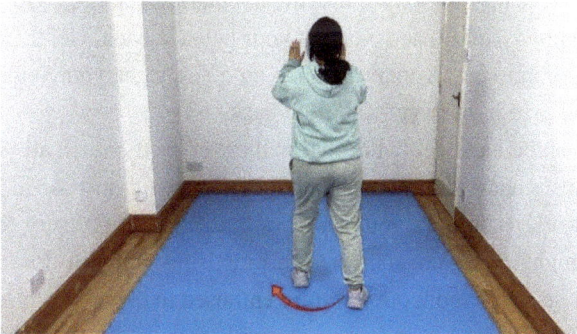

And once more takes you to the other side.

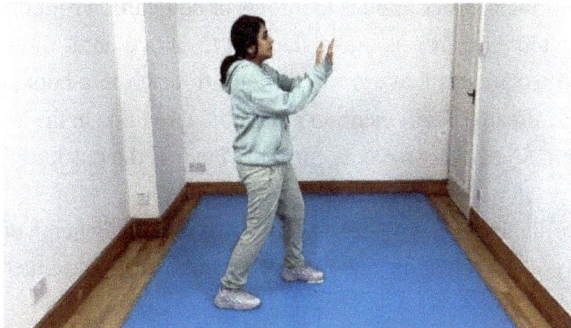

Practice this both ways. Going clockwise and also anti-clockwise.

Also practice it mixed with the other footsteps too. Make up your own variations but here are a few you could copy to get the idea. Repeat each of these a few times. They're good for you!

Step forward fully once and now pivot clockwise. Go forwards a step and pivot anti-clockwise.

Now go back first then pivot clockwise. Back and anti-clockwise.

Two steps forwards and then pivot clockwise. Two back and anti-clockwise.

Take two steps to the left and two back after that. Take two steps to the right and two back after that.

You get the idea. You are now moving about in a safe way. Soon get your training partner to pressure you. Maybe get them to pressure you into a corner or up against a wall and you have to find your way out using footwork. Again, you can do this on your own. Get yourself into a corner, imagining someone pressuring you, and then make your way out of there, and fight them off with some Palm Heels.

As you develop this skill of moving about, quicken it up. Get your partner to give you a shove (safely) and you get your balance back. Get them to pull you as if they are going to drag you away, and you quickly get your Wide Fence and get this footwork and base so you can fight back.

So this is the basic footwork that will cover pretty much all you need. It will help you do so many things much better than if you didn't use it. There are more fancy footwork techniques you can learn but it's not necessary for self defence, though it might keep you interested in practising and will do no harm to your abilities, so do check more out if you're enthused to do so. But this is basically all you need. Do practice it and come up with more step and pivot combinations yourself. There are many more!

There are also more elements and applications of balance than just footwork. It's a major principle that applies to throws or being thrown, applies to fighting on the ground too but that is now starting to move into more advanced and complicated techniques that are too difficult to teach in a book, and this book is long enough already. I will mention a little bit about this in the Sensitivity section of The Magic Five otherwise it is currently beyond the reach of this book.

Next we'll move into another principle that will really help you use less energy during a physical altercation and make you much much 'stronger' at pretty much everything you do!

STRUCTURE (FRAMES)

Structure is what makes you so much stronger at everything. Buildings have solid structures to hold them up, so do bridges, so do cars, and so do we. With the correct structures you become much stronger in any given place or situation and you often don't even need to use much strength.

Structure is sometimes called 'framing' in the martial arts because you're creating a frame with your body, though you won't hear the term used very much.

Structure applies in so many places but you already know some of these. The best structure for when you're standing up - The Fence! And the best structure to push back with - the Wide Fence! You already know the best position on the ground too.

I don't want you to be overwhelmed with information here. In my normal teaching I just add this information as we go along and so it fits in seamlessly and you don't have to think about it. But here we have had to learn the skills first and now we are going back to look at them to add The Magic Five. We are having to break things down more than I normally would because of this info being in a book. So if it's too much to take in and understand right now, just have a glance through and come back another time. Let it all sink in by itself without extra effort on your behalf. You will pick it up at your own pace.

I have to show you this as it is so integral to you having massive ability and using the least amount of energy as you go through a physical confrontation. So this information is crucial to take you many steps higher but take your time getting there. Most people don't know any of this but you will.

Let's have a look at positions you already know and see how they can actually be made stronger with a little better understanding. Take your time and try out each of these positions. Get in them and have a good think and feel where the structures are strongest and where they can be improved.

So here we are using the Get Up against someone who it between our legs. In this position keeping both your arms solid, along the lines shown in the picture, gives you maximum power and you don't need to use much strength and energy.

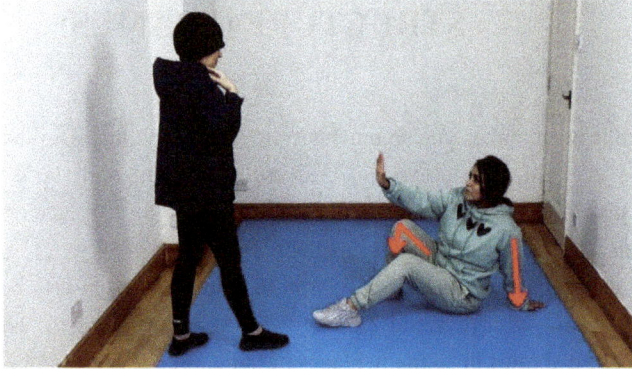

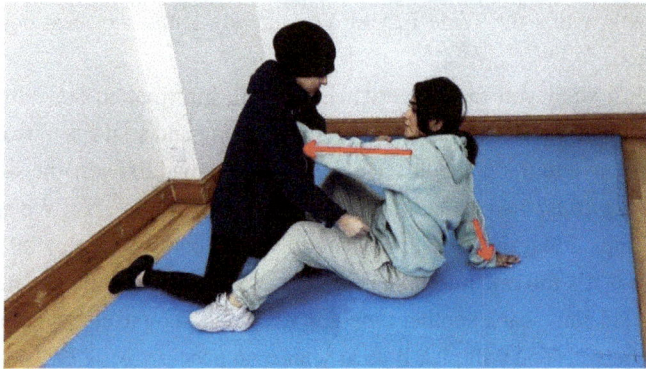

Have a go at this. Remember that you would use this for any time you have fallen to the ground. Here it is being used again to get up off the ground. This time the arrows show the right leg and the left arm as being the structures you need to focus on as those are what you will use to get up. Move your planted foot and arm about a bit to see where they are strongest and where you would use the least strength. Tip: the more vertical they are the stronger they will be. The more diagonal they are the weaker they will be. But this will also depend on your anatomy so you might not be flexible enough to get so vertical with them. But try, then practice the Get Up from the different frames you create.

If you find yourself in this position below, the bent legs and arms will help to hold him off. Of course this is all dynamic and you have to scrap. But using this structure will stop him from getting at you that time.

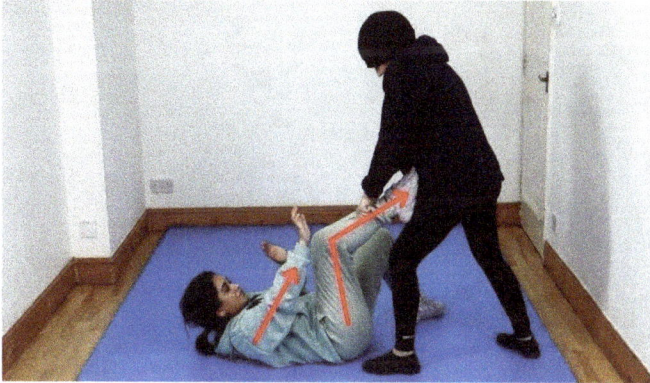

Here the Stiff Arm is combined with the leg pressing down. Your effort travels from your leg and into your arm. Just using your straight arm here requires strength. But if you are more sideways and pushing with your right leg especially you will get more strength going through your right arm. You can use this same structure in pretty much any position when you're underneath.

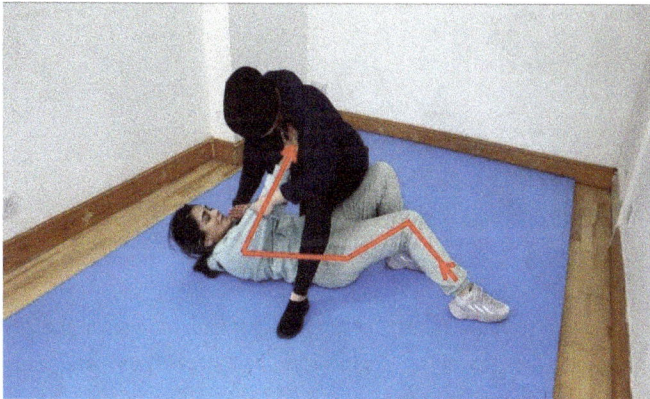

Here is the Strongest Position on The Floor (still doesn't have a name yet, unless I've just named it!). The square you create with your arm can be used to hold him off or to push him.

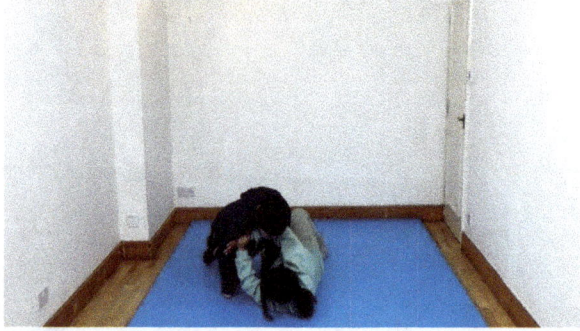

Just note that again you are driving through your leg and then using that energy to drive your arms. Just using your arms will be a lot weaker.

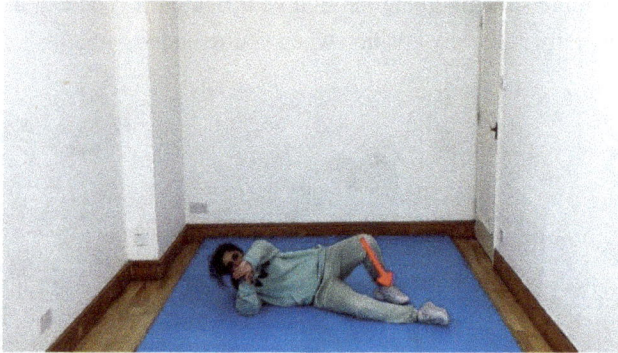

This is another type of frame you might use when you are on the ground. Your legs bent provide the power to Bridge too so you can push and slide out from underneath when you create space.

Your arms press ups against both his and you use the strength of your legs

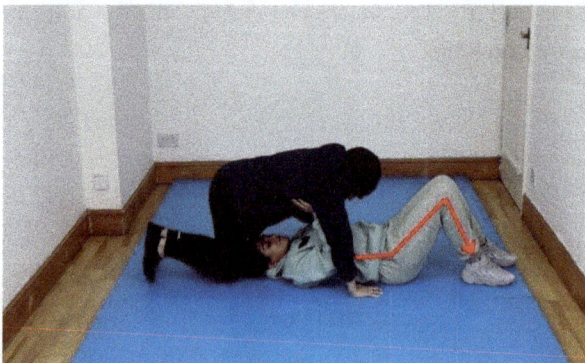

(and the Bridge) to allow you to breathe if he's smothering you. You might be able to push him off too from here.

The Stiff Arm is also a frame. Don't just push with your arm. You push with your whole body while it is a solid frame. Now he's coming up against the pressure of your body pushing him and not just the strength of your iddly widdly little tricep muscle.

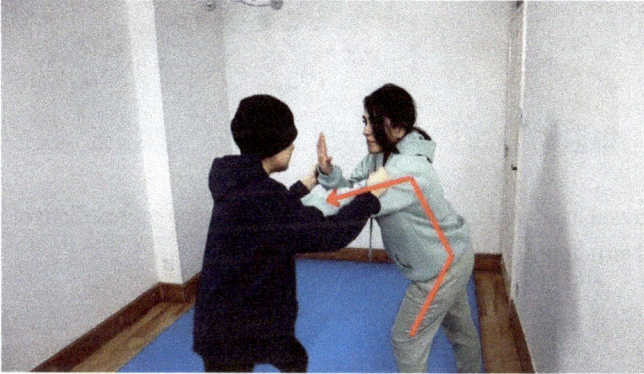

Here you are using various frames to keep him from scooping you up or dragging you to the floor etc.

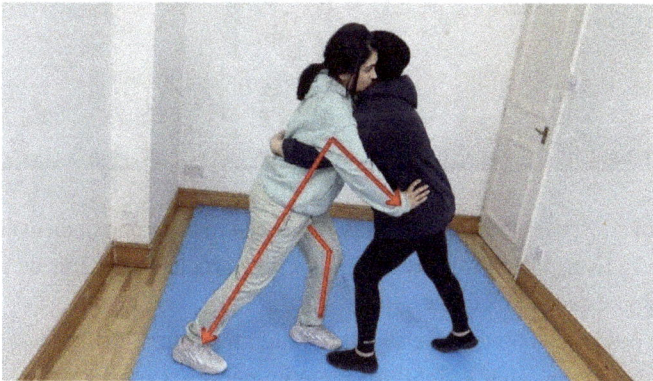

And here again in the bear hug from the rear you are using a frame to create a relatively safe place to start working from. Having that strong frame is what causes him to struggle to deal with you the way he wants.

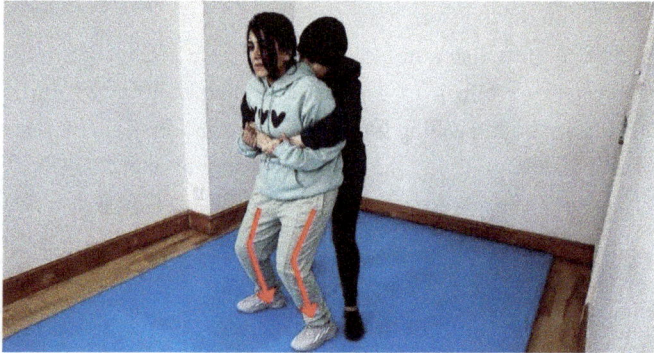

The clawed hand you use for scratching is also much more effective if you see it as a solid structure.

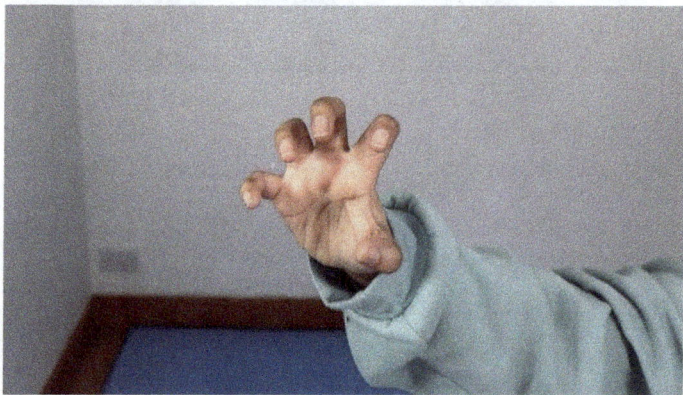

The Covert Fences too are structures. You need to be strong in them and ready for an attack. Even if you're playing it cool, the structure needs to be ready, to resist being grabbed for example.

Where possible you must use structure rather than strength. The less strength you use as you go through a fight, the more immensely strong you'll seem. And you'll last longer and the more he'll wonder why when he's pushing you in the fight you're not struggling as much as you should be.

With good structures you use less energy overall and so won't be out of breath as much.

So wherever you are, try to think of where the structure is in what you're doing. Can you create a strong frame which to work from? Usually you can.

You already know some of the most powerful frames. When you go through this book and try things again, now focus on making them into frames that you will work from, and suddenly all these positions have become even stronger than before and you'll be using less energy to fight from them! Isn't that amazing?!

Now you are really taking things to another level.

But we haven't finished yet! We've got a few more enhancers we can add.

CENTRE OF MASS

The Centre of Mass is located just below your bellybutton at the navel and it's where your bodyweight is balanced. The central location around where your whole bodyweight is and where gravity has the most influence. Around there anyway. Of course it varies a little for all of us and men tend to be top heavy and so their centre of mass is a little closer to the bellybutton. Women are generally lower-half heavy and so have a slightly lower centre of mass, but really it's not a massive enough difference for us to be concerned. The actual location of the centre of mass is halfway between your back and your front, inside your body, but for our purposes we can keep things simple and think of it as being at about the navel.

For the purposes of self defence we are going to use centre of mass, centre of gravity and centre of balance interchangeably to mean just one thing. Now, just in case you're a physicist and are about to throw your Van De Graaf generator at this book in anger, hold on to your Bunsens while I explain. I know they are different things, and not interchangeable in physics. But for our current purposes I am just going to refer to it as centre of mass although I might technically be wrong at some points and you, as a physicist, might be tutting.

All we really need to know for self defence is this area (the centre of mass/navel area) needs to be controlled if we want to generate maximal forces with our body.

Another way to think of this area is that it is the hips. If you move that whole area (the hips) solidly you will generate more forces. Like, massively more forces. (Combine this with your knowledge of Structure and Balance and now you're in some serious power-generating territory, using physics, maths and biomechanics to assist you. And we haven't finished with the Magic Five yet. There's still two more!).

So, I know I'm telling you how to find this area in several different ways but it's very important. Being able to use your centre of mass just makes everything better. Makes you hit harder, push harder, pull harder. It makes you resist forces better.

You knew I was going to say that! I said it with the two previous principles of The Magic Five too!

But that is actually a major premise of this book, and what I teach. Not just show a few techniques that work in the real world but take them several levels higher to make them even more effective, preferably stopping every altercation as soon as it starts. We want him to hit a wall as soon as he starts anything. We must prepare for the worst but we train so we never get there.

The thing is that each of these Magic Five enhances you in a slightly different way, though each of them genuinely adds serious clout to what you're doing overall.

From a training point of view, remember you can add these one at a time. You don't have to learn them all today. This book is for long term development if you want it. So you can come back and add the Magic Five one at a time, in your own time. But the sooner you do, the sooner you will be more able!!

Centre of Mass was one of the first sports principles I discovered and learned a very long time ago when I was still a kid. It added so much power to my striking ability that I've always been one of the hardest hitters in any gym or dojo I ever went to. It was knowing and applying this principle that allowed me to generate this impressive power.

However, with regard to hitting, there is a caveat. You can only hit as hard as your body can take. Only as hard as your bones and tendons and muscles can handle. So you are limited as to how hard you can hit. The stronger all bones and tendons and muscles are, the harder you can hit. That's obvious, right?

The Palm Heel again wins out with regards to this. Due to the way you mechanically use your body, everything is aligned better and so you rely less on muscles bones and tendons as you're actually using more of a frame to hit with rather than strength.

We have already dealt with some aspects of Centre of Mass already with regards Bad Guy trying to pick you up or push you about. So I'm just going to remind you and this time also say that apart from having a good structure to fight from, now start thinking about using the Centre of Mass in a more active and dynamic role.

Think about where you can use Centre of Mass in all that you've learned so far.

The way you use the Centre of Mass is really simple:

In any direction that you want to generate a force, just move your centre of mass in that direction.

That's it. It really is as simple as that but might require a little bit of adjustment to make it work for you if you're not used to the principle.

So going back to him trying to push or pull you about, get your partner to do it again, but this time focus on really resisting from the Centre of Mass.

So stand up and let your training partner first pull you as if they're going to drag you away. But you resist like before, only this time you need to bring your hips into the equation.

Have a think. In which direction do you need to move your hips (generate forces) to resist the pull? Yep, it's backwards and downwards. So that's the direction you need to move your Centre of Mass to create maximum force that way. Try it. Just see how much stronger you have suddenly become and how little strength you have to use to do this rather than trying to fight your way through using strength.

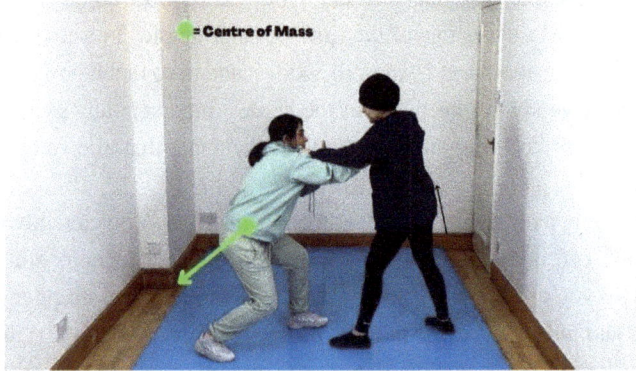

In this same position, now get you partner to push you (last time they pulled). Now you push back whilst employing the Centre of Mass as you do so. You will find that you can't be pushed so easily. You have just massively improved your ability to not get shoved or dragged about!

In fact, get your partner to stand and give them a push, if it safe to do so and you've discussed it with each other. You don't need to push them off the surface of the earth. You're just going to try something. First push them as you would normally and note what the results are. Second time push whilst engaging your navel area, which you might need to tense up a bit as you push. Now see how much harder they were pushed. Let's do a third push. This time I don't even want you to use much effort at all. I want you to use movement to generate the force.

So this time, make sure your Centre of Mass is fully moving in the direction you want to send your training partner.

Note how you don't have to actually move that area much at all to generate massive forces! That's because it is sending your whole bodyweight behind that push. Instead of your muscles pushing him, which let's say is using 20-30 kilos of force, you're now using 50 AND you didn't really use much energy nor muscular strength to do it!

You're starting to become a pretty high level martial artist now! (Whether you wanted to or not!)

There's more going on than just moving your bodyweight. There is also the element which you might remember from physics classes as being called 'momentum'. For our purposes just understand that once you have had a few practices at engaging your hips in pushes and pulls, now you can make your movement sharper and faster. Just add a short sharp push (or pull) to make this whole technique even better. But you can come back and do that later.

So, I've said above that the Centre of Mass has to move in the direction you need to generate the force. That is true, but often you don't even need to move it much at all. Often the tiniest movement in the direction can generate a lot of force. So if someone catches you off guard let's say, you can tense up your navel area and just move it the tiniest amount, just a millimetre, and it will generate a lot of resistance.

So, let's go back to the position above. Your training partner is pulling you and you're resisting. You're leaning fowards as above. Now they switch to pushing you and I want you to resist that immediately by changing the direction your hips are generating force. So now you're pushing back. I want you to do this without moving your hips much at all. Almost as if you are static. Almost as if you did the whole thing inside your head.

Get them to pull again and you can suddenly switch to resisting that and you're strong already! In a millisecond!

Centre of Mass is so important to how you generated those forces and you did it really rapidly and properly powerfully.

You are now becoming really difficult to shove around!

Of course, you still need a solid structure, and you need to keep all the basics, but you can now see how Centre of Mass can help you.

We're going to cover a couple more ways you can use it, but I wanted to point out here that you've actually started using the fourth principle of The Magic Five already too. You've started using Sensitivity. You've started to feel what the other person is doing. Feeling if they're pushing or pulling, and then acting on that. It's like developing a superpower. It's like developing a Spidey-sense. We'll come back to this in the next chapter but I wanted you to be aware of it.

My sister Rahilla and Bad Guy are going to demonstrate a few places where you could now start applying Centre of Mass to do more work for you.

Back to when you were escaping grabs, now when you're knocking someone's gripping hand, coordinate your Centre of Mass with the whacking off of the hand, as shown by the arrow, and you will be SO much stronger in the action. Like, his hand will fly off your wrist if you're doing this properly. If it's not flying off, then keep practising! It can take a second whack to get it off sometimes so do follow up if the first doesn't work. Some people do have very strong grips. But you will be so much better at this if you use your Centre of Mass to whack his hand off.

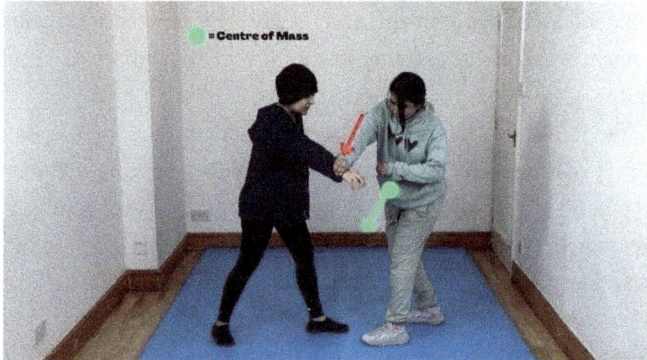

In a kick to the groin, remember we want to kick so hard that he is lifted onto his toes (metaphorically if not in reality). To do that you need your hips to move upwards mostly but with a slight forwards travel too.

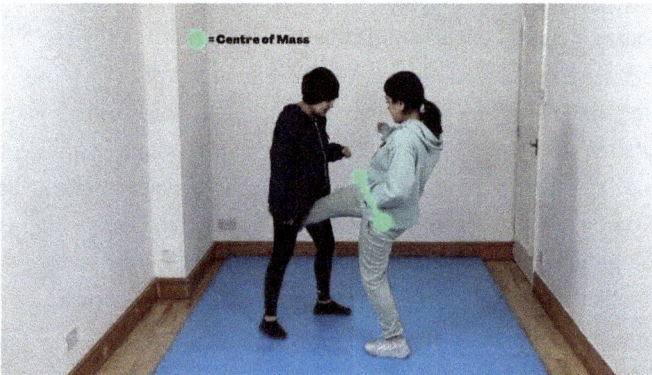

So these are just some examples of where you can add this magical principle and make everything more effective. It works on the floor as much as it works on the ground. When it comes to being thrown, if you drop your Centre of Mass lower than his it becomes very difficult for him to throw you. Actually if you try to throw someone or do a 'takedown' of any kind, you need to get underneath their Centre of Mass and then control it. In fact, if you're on the floor with him on top, have a think where his Centre of Mass is and if you can just push really hard at that spot. You might find he either just falls off (and you scramble up) or you'll find he loses enough balance to create a gap or weakness that you can slide out through.

It is just so universally applicable and such a useful concept to use in self defence.

From a sports point of view it is also one of the most useful things you can know about. If you play tennis or you do the long jump or even if you canoe or do any other sports activity, have a think about where your Centre of Mass is and how you might be able to use it. I bet it will enhance pretty much every sport that you take part in! Even if you're using a hammer whilst you're building a shed, or you really want to slam a door shut so somebody knows about it, use your Centre of Mass to help you make it into a more powerful and effective move, whilst actually using less energy to do so!

One more of The Magic Five coming up next!

SENSITIVITY

You must have heard the 'use his strength against him' idea from the martial arts?

This is it!

Rickson Gracie (have I mentioned him before!) calls this 'feel'. He says, "Feel what is going on, don't think."

Some others call it 'connection', some call it feel but 2.5 decades back, when I first learned this principle, it didn't have a name so I called it 'Sensitivity'. Hopefully you'll see why, but you can call it whatever you prefer.

I learned it from a world rated Aikido competitor whilst I worked in a gym in Hammersmith, London. I'm going to call this guy 'Dave' though that was not his real name. Dave was a regular attendee at the gym but we never really crossed paths, just nodded heads in passing. He was then involved in a major motorbike accident where his hands were literally shredded in some places. He was told he would never use his hands properly again. He was wearing protective leather gloves at the time of the accident but that's motorbike accidents for you. I've attended quite a few in my time in the police and they're not all that pleasant to deal with.

As Dave was trying to recover, continuously having surgery after surgery to adjust things as much as possible, he wanted to keep his martial arts game up. He'd never have trained with someone as low down the food chain as me but now he was badly injured and needed someone to work with he could trust. I was there at the gym all the time and he'd heard I was a martial artist though not ranked at anything so it was just convenient to train with me. He was ten years my senior and a training nut like I was so I happened to be in the right place at the right time and now I found myself being personally coached by him.

He didn't know but I had my own specialities. I might not have been a competitive fighter but I knew a fair amount of boxing and something new I had discovered from a self defence legend named Geoff Thompson (the person who named and developed The Fence - and certified me as an coach one day much later). I was learning ground grappling and how to fight on the ground. It was my speciality and very few people actually knew anything about it at the time. This was in the mid 90's and the jiu jitsu craze hadn't started yet. It was just called 'ground grappling' or 'ground-fighting' and to this Aikido man it was something totally new and out of his experience.

There was nowhere near to train ground fighting at the time so I'd learned it from books and videos and then practised with a few friends I'd found across the width of London. Learning it involved a lot of travel at the time because so few places coached it or knew anything about it. Dave was a ranked competitor in Aikido before his injury, had a black belt in judo and was a good Muay Thai kickboxer. I was good at punching; he was good at kicking. He was good at throwing; I was good on the ground. He was doing competitive martial arts with rules and regulations; I was learning self defence where we only applied rules as we saw fit for training so we didn't damage our training partner. We were literally doing the opposite of each other at everything! So his areas of strength were my areas of weakness and my areas of strength were his areas of weakness.

This was another lucky streak in my life. So we both held back our egos and coached each other several times a week.

One of the first things he taught me, a major staple in Aikido, is to use your enemies energy against them. So I was lucky to learn this principle at a very early stage in my martial arts and I've been applying it to everything since then. It is one of the reasons why other martial artists always tell me that I'm very strong, even when I know that I'm not.

No matter where I went, and what I learned, I always applied this principle and it made me feel to them that I was stronger than I actually was. And that's what it will do for you.

So, to finish the story about my Aikido friend, we coached each other whilst his hands improved over the next year or more. He wanted to get fit, defy the doctors and train fully because they'd said he never would. You'll be glad to know he did prove them wrong by about 90%.

Anyway, I have never had this principle clarified to me anywhere else and I've not seen it coached anywhere else. That's why I've not ever known what it is called, though I'm sure in Aikido they probably have a name for it. The only time I've heard anyone name it was two years ago when I heard Rickson talking about this concept and he called it 'Feel'. But I was already stuck on the name 'Sensitivity'. So you call it what you like. But I bet you'd heard of the principle, didn't know what it's called and had no real idea what it is or how to use it. But you've already been introduced to it in this book and actually even had a few practices at it.

The first thing to understand is that you can only really use Sensitivity when the person touches you, connects any part of their body to yours. If you are not touching then Sensitivity does not apply.

Sensitivity is body awareness - yours and theirs - feeling where they're applying pressure - pulling or pushing or lifting or dropping or twisting. What are they contacting with? Their chest? Their legs? Their hands?

And how much pressure are they applying?

Where is their bodyweight?

And can you use all that against them.

So let's go back a little to the previous chapter where your partner was pushing you and you were using your Centre of Mass. You can try this now with your training partner if you like. As they push you can actually feel them doing that. At first resist them from moving you.

But what if you suddenly stopped resisting and moved out of the way? They would go flying past you!

Now you are starting to use sensitivity. Starting to use their own strength against them.

Hey, how about as they're going flying past, you give them a bit of a shove too? Just a tiny shove, because this is training.

But what you will see is that even with a tiny shove, they're going to fly even further than they were originally.

And here's the best thing - they think you did all that, sent them flying, because you have the strength of She-Hulk.

So that, in its basic essence is how you use the other person's strength against them. Grappling martial artists use this all the time but most don't actually know it as conscious principle. They do it because they've done it for so long and their brain has just learned to do it. But once it becomes a conscious thing you can really use it right away, without years of training, and you can choose to apply it to so many places, especially escaping from someone holding you, or throwing them etc.

Let's say someone is sitting on top of you in the Full Mount. You can feel where their weight is. You can feel where they are pressing and also where they are very light. Remember we have actually done this earlier in the chapter on ground escapes.

All this is usable information. You can actually feel all this with your eyes closed. Try it. Just feel where he is pushing or pulling, in which direction and with what quantity of force.

And you can fight against, push or pull, and slip out of where he is lightest. Or you can throw him off you if you feel where he is balanced at his weakest.

If you are flat on the floor, face down, and Bad Guy is getting onto your legs or back, you can feel where he is and thus turn appropriately to deal with him.

If someone is trying to push you off a balcony or against a wall, you can feel where they are weakest and slide out that way. Or you could just push back for a second so they push harder, then you suddenly release all that, move out of the way and let them fly off the balcony themselves, while you head away to have a croissant and a coffee and call the police.

If someone has pushed you against a wall or into the corner of a wall, feel where they are weakest, and escape that way. If they're not giving you much force to work with, push them, pull them and you'll see they react and start giving you forces to play with.

Sensitivity is a super important skill enhancer. Even if you're not using proper skills and techniques it will still enhance what you do.

And you know what?

It's probably too difficult to teach it in a book!

But I hope you've learned something and it didn't just appear as gobbledegook. For the moment, when you are training with a partner, just start feeling where they are pressuring and where they are not. And use that against them. They'll suddenly think you've got the strength of King Kong!

BODY MECHANICS

This is the fifth, but by no means least, of The Magic Five. It has equal weighting to the others as a technique and power enhancer.

Once more I'll to try to explain something that's not so easy to do in a book but would be unfair to keep out. I believe I can explain the concept enough that you can use it but it's too difficult to show how to apply it to everything. It applies to so many techniques and situations though it is more detailed, technical and nuanced than the other four Magic enhancers. But I'll have a go at it and hopefully this will help you.

Body Mechanics (my own term again) is the ability to use as much of your body as you can to do an action.

So let's say you're going to use a hammer and chisel to create a beautiful ice sculpture. It's going to be the head and shoulders of Nefertiti. You have the hammer in your hand and the chisel blade resting on the block of ice. You want nice delicate forces to craft the intricacies of her headgear and necklaces and eyes and face. So you use the movement of your wrist and a little movement from your elbow too. Be careful though! Don't break too much off!

So you created this beautiful Nefertiti, everyone loved and admire it, but and it's the end of the show and now you have to smash her to bits. You need to make her into ice cubes for the afterparty.

To smash the sculpture you will need a big swing of the hammer. You'll need to make sure your wrist and elbow is really working hard for starters. What about the shoulder? If you want to hit hard and get those ice cubes for your fruit cocktails you now have to add power and speed and swing from the shoulders too.

You're starting to get the job done and the sculpture will be gone in no time, leaving you with only with refreshments and memories.

For self defence there is rarely going to be a time you want to be delicate. We have to be able to smash that hammer, get it to cause destruction, preferably the very first time we strike it. We don't want to make Nefertiti from that block. We want to make ice cubes.

This is what Body Mechanics is for our purposes. Using as much of your body as you can to do the job.

Now, Body Mechanics is one of the places where women tend to differ a lot from men. In general, women use much less of their body to do an activity. A woman throwing a ball for example, will do so using her wrist, elbow and a little bit of her shoulder and that's about it. She won't throw with her whole body. I say this anecdotally, though it's from decades of experience teaching sports. Of course not all women do this. But women do have a greater tendency to do it than men. I want to make sure you're aware of it as it could really determine a lot of your power output. I don't know what the reason for this is but if I were to guess, then I think the reason could be how girls and boys are brought up differently. It appears that women can move mechanically correctly. For example female tennis players or athletes use their whole bodies in their jobs. Professional boxers do too and so on. So it's not something that women cannot do, but I have noticed it as something that does happen more regularly in women. I don't say this to offend or cause controversy or anything like that. I just want to make sure that this is highlighted so you have the option of paying more attention to this area if you want to. It may be something you are not aware you do and so this knowledge will assist you greatly.

Now, back to the the ice smashing, or even the ball throwing. If you added the top of your spine, say at about where the sternum is, and also employed this area to generate forces, you're now going to generate even more.

So now you're using your wrist, elbow, shoulder and also moving the area at about your sternum too.

Let's say you did all this during a Palm Heel or elbow or even a punch, you will be generating some very interesting forces.

But that's not even enough! The spine moves at each of the vertebrae. You've already engaged the area at the sternum and it is moving. Next you need to focus on just below that. Where your six-pack lies. If you crunch all that area when you Palm Heel or throw or push, you're now going to add even more power to what you're doing.

Try it out. You can do it in a couple of ways. If you have a partner with pads to hit or if you have a punching bag to hit, then start the Palm Heel with just your elbow doing the work. Next add the shoulder. Then the upper part of your torso is added to push forwards. Then your six-pack area. You will see and feel how much more force you're generating and you won't be using much more energy to create this extra power. You are using the mechanics of your body. (This is actually part of 'biomechanics' in sport science but I don't use that term for my own teaching purposes as it encompasses far more than we need for self defence).

So Body Mechanics is the ability to employ more of your body to do a physical task.

Try it in other ways too. If you don't have a partner to practice Palm Heels, you can actually just stand facing a wall, put your hand onto the wall, and then try all of the above. You're actually doing more of a push now than Palm Heels, but having a good push is also very useful for self defence. You could practice it with both hands and find you are going to be able to push so much harder. (Add Centre of Mass to that and see what that does too!)

So push only with your wrist. Next emphasise the elbow too. Then the shoulder, and then the upper torso and then the lower. You'll see how much more powerful you are but without really using much more energy.

Next time you're in need of hammering something, think about this. Or when you're throwing a ball and need it to travel a fair distance, think about this.

The same is applicable if you're resisting someone pushing you or if you're kicking something. Like kicking the car tyre when you break down whilst you head to the beach on your only weekend off in the summer. You will be able to kick that tyre much harder if you use Body Mechanics, though, thinking about it, maybe you shouldn't use Body Mechanics on this occasion. Just call the repair van.

There is more to Body Mechanics than is stated here, and like I said, I tend to incorporate it into everything I teach so it's always applied and makes you stronger at everything that you do. So, like with the rest of The Magic Five, start incorporating this into your own training and add it as extra knowledge. I want you to employ a lot of your body when you're doing a technique. Embed this idea into your training and start using it soon. Maybe even go through the book again and apply it to all the skills there.

It is the use of these Magic Five concepts that will help you to be less tired throughout a situation and to be pushing around the Bad Guy rather than the other way round. These are the things that will really add to your ability to stop him early because he's going to be hitting a brick wall every time he tries something. The Magic Five really are quite super and I hope I have demonstrated to you how truly effective they are and why you should practice them.

For a very long time, while I went the route of competing in martial arts, I never told them to anyone except family, very close friends and a tiny selection of people I trained. But if you'd ever met me in the training arena you'd know there was something different going on, that I was really quite strong and immovable when I wanted to be. Other competitors thought it was strength but it was these skills I've walked you through combined with the basic skills. That was it.

And now you know them too. Don't tell anyone else about them, please!!

IN CONCLUSION

When I started the journey of writing this book I thought I should first check out the 'competition'. See what they'd written.

What competition? There wasn't any! There were a few pamphlet's out there throwing out a few techniques but nothing substantial.

It's hard to write a book! You have to do plenty of research and analysis. It's like putting together a giant jigsaw where all the pieces are in your head and you have to keep searching for them in there somewhere. (Have I already mentioned the brain damage I'm getting from writing this?!) Apparently only clever people can write and finish books but that wasn't going to stop me!

I thought I'd check to see what online courses there were. I found less than a handful but honestly it was the same thing - men's self defence that women were allowed. They didn't cover the necessary skills specifically for women. I knew it was unlikely anyone had a strategy to deal with a man following a woman because that was something quite unique to my experience. It had come about through necessity and unless someone else had the same needs it was unlikely they'd have developed a solution for a man approaching from behind.

But it wasn't only that which was lacking but most other things too. There was literally no psychological or mindset input. Just pure physical techniques, dumped onto a page. No coherence or progression or development for the reader/student. This is just wrong in my eyes! Isn't the job of a coach to ensure the student develops? Did I get this wrong. Is the job of the coach to just dump a pile of info and let them work it out for themselves? I didn't think so. Maybe I took my job too seriously.

Anyway, all sports people will tell you that the psychological aspects of sport are equally as important as the physical and tactical. But in self defence situations, they are *super* important. Your life could be on the line. That is a mental challenge more than even a physical one. Of course you must have the physical skills to protect your life and limbs, but, unlike a competitive athlete in sports or the martial arts, you can't walk away from your situation. When you're in it you have to deal with it. And it's the mental game that you need to have control of throughout if you want to survive. You have to know what the person is going to do, how he will approach you, how he will deceive you. You need to know how to generate anger to beat freeze. You have to know that persistence is what wins a fight in the end. And you have to apply these mental skills throughout, which is why I urge you to go over them again several more times. It is only through repetition that you will really understand them and make them practical and usable. Craft your own notes about them, if you like. Even practice and rehearse the psychology, visualise it. Take from this book what suits you best. Only you know what you really need and you can always come back another time to go over things again.

Back to what I was saying. Nobody covered mindset anywhere. It was only the physical techniques - most of which are quite ineffective and untested in reality, telling women to trip a man to the floor and fight him there and suchlike, as if the real world is the same as the dojo. Just silliness.

But the thing that really annoyed me the most, and one of the reasons I was fretting to write this book, is how kickboxing, Krav Magaga and Gracie jiu jitsu are sold as self defence.

I saw women ask the question on online forums, "what self defence should I do?" The answer was usually one of these three. Sometimes it was something else but these are the flavour of today and it genuinely angered me that this advice was given again and again because it's the wrong advice and will get people hurt or even killed.

But I think people just don't know. They weren't purposely handing out bad advice. They believed they were genuinely helping. There are no other books out there like this one, written by someone who's trained martial arts for an infinity, who also had to test all those skills against some big bad wolves in London, and has spent at least two thirds of his life in one sport or another. Did I mention I had a degree in Sport Science as well? And most people aren't self defence crazy like some of us - and so maybe they just don't really understand what self defence is. They were giving out the best advice they could at the time.

But that advice really needs correcting, because it will save lives if the truth is out there.

And so now I can stop seething at Reddit and Facebook responses to the question of what martial art women should do for self defence. The answer is…they should do self defence for self defence. So read this book!

I hope you realise that what's in this book makes more sense than learning flying kicks and strangling someone with their own shoelaces. That you need to keep your feet on the ground and that you're not a ninja who needs to stay and fight to the death. I hope what you have read (and practiced!) makes legitimate sense and you know what a woman or girl needs to know if she wants to know self defence that is universally applicable. These skills stand the test of time. They won't change until men grow a second head, at which time you might not need these skills anyway because those prone to attacking women might stop when they grow an extra brain, right?

The thing is that martial arts do work, including kickboxing, Krav Maga and jiu jitsu. They work because they provide the practitioner with a heightened sense of confidence. Confidence is the queen of all sports, including martial arts and self defence. Confidence gets you to places way beyond what a lack of it would do. Confidence oozes from every pore when you have it. The Bad Guy can see it from a mile away, smell it from a distance and he hates it. He hates it because he knows he's got a battle on his hands and all he wanted was to get his way.

He only wanted you to let him do what he wanted and it now looks like he's not going to get it all easily.

The martial arts give this confidence and luckily their skills rarely get tested in the real world.

So even if you didn't read all the chapters or maybe didn't actually practice everything suggested, get yourself a tonne of confidence. Get it in bucket-loads. It's the first thing the attacker sees and he doesn't like it.

But if you did actually go through the book then you should have the genuine confidence that these are the skills that will work for you if you ever needed them, tried and tested.

I hope you got your own take-aways from the book. If you think it could benefit your friends or family or colleagues, then please do let them know about it. You could mention us to your welfare officer or senior leader at work or university/college school and we may be able to teach your organisation online or in person. So please do refer us forwards if you think that is something appropriate to do.

Finally, if you don't mind, just for the last few seconds, I'd like to reiterate what you should have learned if I've done my job correctly:

You should have learned...

... that he ain't no monster. No matter how horrible he is, he's only a man. So we can do things to him.

If you're scared. That's good.

Get angry. It will focus you. He has no right to harm or invade your life. You didn't give him permission to do that.

So get angry if you're scared.

And walk away if you can. Get to a safer place if you can. Find help if you can.

You might not even have to fight!

If you have to fight, keep your Fence up and work from there. The Fence is magic in itself. It can stop things before they start, and it will have you ready for anything that comes your way. So get up your Fence!

Still try to get away if you can. Still continue being loud. Still look for help and ways out.

Then stay on your feet. Get Up if you are on the floor.

Keep disobeying. Keep disengaging. Get your distance and keep moving away.

Fight him off when you have to.

Keep shouting and BE LOUD! Project your voice across the hills and far away so everyone can hear you then call the rescue squads. Put hard heat on this man so he runs away like the pathetic mouse that he really is.

Repeat everything if you have to.

And if you're in real danger…

Get mad! Get visceral.

The animal inside will save you.

Make him unconscious. Send him back to his Maker if that's what you need to do.

But at all costs, YOU have to win.

To live.

To walk away and drink coffee and have cake.

That is self defence.

You know it. And now you have the skills to back it up.

So, peace, take care of your loved ones and yourselves. I am ecstatic to be of service to you. All the best from me.

I'm off now to munch chocolate macarons with some tea. Please don't tell my mother! I'm not allowed too many sweets. She's not here though so maybe I'll have a vanilla slice? I could decide at the patisserie... probably end up having a doughnut as I haven't kicked that habit since the police and there really is a FANTASTIC doughnut shop in York...

Uh oh! I'm talking to myself again... You've already left to practice!

See you around! Ciao, for now!

Hafiz Younis.
BSc (Hons) Sport Science.
Chief Coach at Power For Women.

HELPFUL RESOURCES

The Samaritans
Provide 24/7 confidential & emotional support for anyone experiencing despair, distress or suicidal feelings.
Tel: 116123 (free). www.samaritans.org jo@samaritans.org Text: 077725909090

National Domestic Abuse Helpline
Run in partnership with Women's Aid & Refuge. www.nationaldahelpline.org.uk
Tel: 0800 2000 247

Rights of Women
Provides women with free, confidential legal advice by specialist women solicitors & barristers. Tel: 020 725 8887 (Tue Only 11-1pm) www.rightsofwomen.org.uk
info@row.org.uk

The Havens
(specialist sexual assault referral centres). Based in London but will speak to everyone.   Tel: 020 3299 6900   www.thehavens.org.uk

Clare's Law
Domestic Violence Disclosure Scheme (DVDS). This is a policy giving women the right to know if their current or ex-partner has any previous history of violence or abuse. www.clares-law.com

Sarah's Law
Child Sex Offender Disclosure Scheme. This Scheme allows parents, carers or guardians to formally ask the police for information about a person who has contact with their child, or a child close to them, if they're concerned the person may pose a risk. www.gov.uk/guidance/find-out-if-a-person-has-a-record-for-child-sexual-offences

Police Crime Stats
This site provides reported crime statistics for UK areas. This can be used to help you plan when you move home or when you apply for jobs etc. Worth a browse.
www.police.uk/search?q=Crime+statistics

Sane

Deals with all aspects of mental illness including depression, anxiety and schizophrenia. Tel: 0845 767 8000. www.sane.org.uk

Mind

Information, advice, guidance and support for people with mental health problems. Tel: 0300 123 3393   email: info@mind.org.uk

Galop

Emotional and Practical support especially for LGBT people experiencing domestic violence. tel: 0800 999 5428. email: help@galop.org.uk

Staying Safe

(from suicidal thoughts) Resources   http://stayingsafe.net

Rethink Mental Illness

Offers Help & Support for those with mental illness
Tel: 0300 5000 927

Papyrus, UK

HOPELineUK is a helpline service giving support & practical advice to under 35s having thoughts of suicide or someone who is concerned about a young person. Tel: 0800 068 4141. Text: 07786 209697

If there are any additions or amendments you think should be in future editions of this book, please let us know via our website. You will be doing everyone a service and your good deed will count for a long time and could help save lives. Peace and health to you.

www.power-for-women.org

ABOUT THE AUTHOR

A brief history of Hafiz Younis ("Everyone calls me "Fizz")

Hafiz wasn't born in the UK. He arrived when he was 3 years old, from Kashmir, which is an interesting place to say the least. The British, the Chinese, the Persians and the Greeks are just some of the people who made their home there at one time or another.

He was lucky enough that his grandfather had been in the British Indian Navy many moons ago and had now invited him over along with his mother and younger brother. He was lucky enough that his father and grandfather chose a very bad town to live in, but he was even more lucky when they chose the worst area of that town and also managed to find the worst street too. That was very lucky and a very interesting way to grow up, considering this was during the 70's and the skinheads and National Front were very popular in Britain at the time. He was about 7 the first time someone spat on his face and told him he was different and that they were going to beat him to death because of that difference. Thankfully that didn't actually happen otherwise he would have been sad about it. The years went by and Hafiz Younis joined the Royal Air Force cadets. That was also interesting but he had the best time of his life and even decided he was going to join the Royal Marines. University put a stop to that idea. He drifted through various sports facilities in the London boroughs of Richmond Upon Thames and later Hammersmith & Fulham coaching everything from athletics to squash and personal training. He coached self defence for a while, including at some prestigious clubs in London and then joined the police because it was something to do and 9 years wearing sports shorts every day was a bit of a chafe. The police seemed like it would be a real job and that turned out to be too true. Having nearly died in riots and with many close calls over a 14 year period, he knew it was time to choose: should he stay or should he go? It was a clash of thoughts. If he went it was to a world unknown, a totally new direction. But if he stayed it was a world with more of the same, all the way to the very end.

And so he went.

And here he is now where you've found him.

In between all that he was doing martial arts pretty much the whole time (with some of the best people in the world, he'd like to add) and also writing crime novels, which he might one day actually finish. He's got four so far in first and second draft mode, but hasn't everyone else out there too? At least he finished this book.

If you were to ever meet him and ask about how things are, he is very likely to say, "They're very interesting."

That's because that's what he thinks.

www.ingramcontent.com/pod-product-compliance
Lightning Source LLC
Chambersburg PA
CBHW050339270326
41926CB00016B/3522